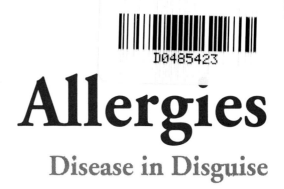

# Allergies
## Disease in Disguise

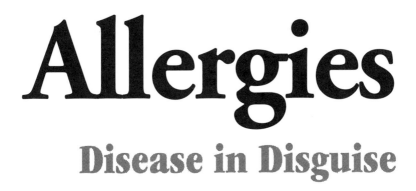

# Allergies
## Disease in Disguise

How to heal your allergic
condition permanently
and naturally

## Carolee Bateson-Koch DC ND

Foreword by Lendon H. Smith MD

**Note to Readers:**
The information in this book is for educational purposes only. It is not intended, and should not be considered, as a replacement for consultation, diagnosis or treatment by a duly licensed health practitioner.

Published by:
Alive Books, 7436 Fraser Park Drive, Burnaby BC Canada V5J 5B9

Illustrations: Janet Sephton
Cover Design: Janet Sephton
Layout & Typography: Sheila Adams

First Printing – February 1994
Second Printing – March 1995


**Canadian Cataloguing in Publication Data**

Bateson-Koch, Carolee, 1942-
Allergies, disease in disguise


Includes bibliographical references and index.
ISBN 0-920470-42-4


1. Allergy—Popular works. 2. Allergy—Treatment—Popular works.
I. Title.
RC584.B37 1994      616.97      C94-910078-1

Printed and bound in Canada.

*To those who are sincerely seeking health.*

# Contents

*Contents*

# List of Figures

# Foreword

*A*bout twenty years ago I began to realize that allergies were causing more than sneezing, wheezing and itching. The parents of my patients were telling me about odd symptoms for which there were no explanations. Emmy got a headache after eating wheat, or Jonathan became hyper if he had orange juice. At first I scoffed at these anecdotal observations because I thought the mothers were trying to avoid blame for some psychological maladjustment. Then when my own children were having odd symptoms that defied a reasonable explanation, I began to believe these reports from many, many patients.

Allergies seemed to be an explanation, so I joined the American College of Allergists. At a meeting I attended in 1970, I was not too surprised to find that there was a schism in the ranks of the members. A new group, the food sensitivity believers, was just forming at that meeting. Dr. James Breneman was the leader of these "radicals." He cited some studies done on bed-wetting that showed that the lining of the bladder in most bed-wetters was speckled with eosinophils, a clear sign of allergy. (That made me feel good because I had been a bed-wetter as a boy and had a son with the problem, which turned out to be a milk sensitivity. No milk, no wet bed. The explanation from psychiatrists was that the child hated the mother and emptied his bladder on the bed – sub-consciously meaning mom.)

In general, however, the group realized they were on shaky ground because there was no test that could clearly distinguish between patients with positive RAST or skin tests and patients with food sensitivities. A reliable, valid, reproducible test would take the anecdotes out of the old wives' category and put food sensitivities into a clinically useful setting. Until recently the only method of diagnosing these food reactions has been presentation of symptoms to a doctor who happened to believe in the reliability of his patient. For example, "After I eat beef (or corn, cheese, soy, peanuts, shellfish, MSG, aspartame, etc.), I feel weak (mean, get a headache, cramps, diarrhea, bloody nose, etc.)."

Doctor's response is, "Don't eat those things." So much for science in the clinical setting. Doctors are loathe to believe that the patient's list of symptoms has any validity without some blood test, X-ray, or palpable lump. When I found food sensitivities in myself and my family that explained mood swings, hyperactivity, bed-wetting, migraines and arthritis, it was easy to find similar reactions in my patients. It was true: anything can do anything.

At that meeting 22 years ago I learned two things: that 80 percent of people with food sensitivities have hypoglycemia, and that food sensitivities cannot do everything, but they can do anything. The standard, traditional allergists are careful to point out that *real* allergies are diagnosed by the RAST (Radioallergosorbent Test) or the skin prick test using extracts. The treatment was to give injections of these antigen-containing extracts in gradually increasing doses to block the allergic reaction.

I thought sugar would be the villain in the hyperactivity scenario, but although that food was part of the picture, it was milk, corn, additives, salicylates, and more importantly, anything the person liked (and craved) that caused of the symptoms. About 60 percent of my hyperactive patients had mood swings and restless behavior if they drank milk. They loved milk. I did tests on these children and discovered they were all low in calcium. No wonder they craved the stuff: they needed the calcium. Apparently, however, no matter how much they drank, it was not absorbed because the intestinal lining cells rejected it. Calcium from other foods plus calcium supplements were necessary to provide helpful therapy for their restless behavior.

I have been delighted with this reassuring, informative, scientifically validated book. It gives me a warm feeling to find a kindred therapist in Dr. Carolee Bateson-Koch. I believe everyone suffers from some food sensitivity. The clues are in this book. Before the reader runs off to the psychiatrist because the doctor can find nothing wrong, the methods outlined in this book should give some relief. Most readers will discover that they are not hypochondriacs or emotional cripples. They are normal human beings forced to breathe polluted air, eat processed food and drink contaminated water.

In summary, the body should be so healthy that digestion will break the ingested foods down into their basic, non-allergic amino acids, fatty acids and simple carbohydrates. It makes sense then, to try to balance the pH of the body, take in nutrient-adequate foods and maintain a low-stress lifestyle. If problems persist, digestive enzyme supplements should help the body maintain homeostasis. We aim for not just health, but robust zest for living.

*Lendon H. Smith, MD*

Lendon H. Smith, MD is the author of:
*Happiness is a Healthy Life, Feed Yourself Right, Feed Your Kids Right, Foods for Healthy Kids, Dr. Lendon Smith's Low Stress Diet, Clinical Guide to the Use of Vitamin C* and *Hyper Kids.*

# Preface

This book is written for my patients, the people who have taught me the most. In return for the privilege of their trust, I wish to provide the specific information they so urgently need in their quest for health.

As a doctor of chiropractic and naturopathy, I have always encouraged questions from my patients. I believe that each patient is entitled to love, respect and answers to his or her questions. I counsel my patients that if a proposed therapy does not seem to follow common sense they should explore it more thoroughly or decline its use. They should understand to the best of their ability whatever therapy they choose, and if their doctor will not answer questions they should choose another doctor.

Over 25 years in practice, it became apparent to me that some other factor was underlying many of the musculoskeletal conditions that I was treating. In searching for answers, I became aware of the involvement of allergy, not only in musculo-skeletal conditions, but in many other conditions as well. Further research confirmed my suspicion that allergy is a serious disease with far-reaching effects – it is much more than just a runny nose. The life-long work of doctors such as Randolph, Rowe and Breneman lends validity to this new and broader concept of allergy.

The incidence of allergic disease is on the rise. In the United States 40 to 50 million people, or one in five adults and children, suffer from allergies. Of these people, 74 percent report that their allergies interfere with work and social life. The most popular methods of fighting allergy – antihistamines and decongestants;

avoiding dust, smoke, pets, perfume and mold; purifying the air – have for the most part been ineffective.

The need for real help for allergic disorders is overwhelming. *Allergies, Disease in Disguise* answers that need. It goes beyond telling the reader how to relieve, manage, control or "attack" allergies: it offers sound, scientific advice and a straightforward method for overcoming allergies.

*Allergies, Disease in Disguise* explains in simple terms how many common health problems are actually allergic disease. This book presents a different view of the process of digestion and how it relates to allergy. It provides a unique treatment plan not found in other books on allergy. That plan includes enzyme therapy – a safe, non-toxic treatment based on scientific research and clinical experience. Additionally, this book describes a new allergic phenomenon, electro-magnetic hypersensitivity syndrome. *Allergies, Disease in Disguise* concludes with an easy, seven step program for complete wellness.

Thousands of people with allergic manifestations are going untreated because the true cause of their symptoms is unrecognized. A goal of this book is to increase public awareness of the scope of allergy so that people can obtain the help they deserve.

## Many thanks to:

*My mother, Dr. Virginia Coffman,*
*for her encouragement, stimulating questions,*
*helpful suggestions and the hard work of proofreading.*

*My husband, Dr. Helmut Koch,*
*for his support, assistance and willingness to discuss ideas.*
*His graciousness was appreciated when time for writing this*
*book interfered with personal and professional schedules.*

*Gisela Temmel, managing editor at Alive Books,*
*for her editing skills, helpful advice, guidance and*
*enthusiasm for this book.*

# 1

# Autobiography of an Allergy

Hello, my name is Al. I'm an allergy. I have a lot of other names too – almost any condition you can name. That's because I'm a great mimicker. I can be anywhere and everywhere in the body and the person doesn't even know I'm there. He or she knows *something* is there, because I can cause pain, discomfort, congestion and other symptoms, but the person doesn't know that it's me, Al the Allergy. He or she thinks I am some other problem and even takes medication for it, but the medication doesn't help. I'm so slick that even the doctors don't recognize me. I'm happiest when I cause inflammation because that's where I like to live, in the midst of warmth, swelling, redness and pain.

Here is the story about where I've been living recently, inside a man I'll call Pete. I gave him a hard time, but he was unusual: he finally caught on that it was me.

Pete was a busy professional and he was well liked by a lot of people. He lived a typical lifestyle for a busy person. He had too many things going on in his life. He worked long hours, didn't get enough rest, went hours without eating, then headed for a restaurant and ate too much, too fast. With this lifestyle plus the demands placed on him by others, his body started to weaken. This is my favorite type. A weakened body allows me to move in, but I do it sneakily. At first I went very slowly so Pete didn't realize anything was going on. I find that when I go slowly enough, the person doesn't notice my presence.

After I had been around for a while, Pete began to have symptoms. First he noticed a rise in blood pressure, then an enormous amount of gas after eating. Yet there was no pain, so Pete didn't do much about it. He took a blood pressure pill.

One morning, after a couple of years, Pete woke up wheezing. This disappeared during the day, so Pete ignored it. I was really sneaky now. Just for good measure, I didn't cause wheezing every day, but only on occasion. That confuses everybody.

Then Pete decided to go hunting. He camped out for a week. The weather was very cold, and one night it snowed. His body was weakened by the cold. Every time he stressed his body, I got a little better foothold and claimed more territory for myself. The wheezing came back worse than ever. About now Pete was getting a little smarter. He took some vitamins and the wheezing went away for a while. So I turned my attention elsewhere.

I can go anywhere in the body, and I found the prostate was a good place to work on next. I stayed there for such a long time that Pete's prostate began to swell bigger and bigger. Pete went to the urologist to have it checked and was told nothing was wrong. I won again. The doctor didn't know that I was there.

Months went by and I was more comfortable than ever. Pete was having more problems. He was running to the bathroom frequently to urinate, especially at night. In the morning, he strained to have a bowel movement. The prostate had enlarged to the point that it was pressing on the rectum, not allowing free passage of the fecal matter. With all the straining at the stool, Pete's blood pressure went even higher. Still, the doctor could find nothing wrong. I chuckled to myself after each trip to the doctor, because my masquerade was still intact. Nobody knows my abilities.

One day Pete had lunch in a local restaurant. He ordered a seafood salad. It was a great opportunity. I already had homes in the intestine, lungs and prostate, but now I could make the one in the intestine better than ever. Within an hour I was at work. Pete noticed the pain about an hour after lunch but he continued to work throughout the afternoon. The pain intensified, and Pete had to take numerous breaks. He managed to get through the afternoon and the pain subsided toward evening.

Pete's wife arrived at the office because they were scheduled to attend a buffet dinner with a group of people from one of the numerous clubs of which Pete was a member. She saw he was pale from the afternoon of pain and suggested they cancel their plans and go home to rest. However, Pete was feeling better now and insisted on attending the event as planned. I was delighted with his decision.

In the middle of the dinner, the pain, now located under Pete's liver, returned so intensely that he was forced to excuse himself. He stumbled out of the restaurant. Unable to drive, he had his wife take him to the nearest hospital emergency room.

At first the doctor investigated for heart problems, thinking that Pete was probably having a heart attack. After ruling that out, he turned his attention to the gall bladder. As this was a Friday night, the doctor scheduled Pete for gall bladder surgery on Monday morning.

The doctor gave Pete some pain killers, but the pain continued throughout the night anyway. By morning Pete was resting better and was no longer in pain. On Sunday Pete was told that the results of all the tests done on him were negative, and that it appeared his gall bladder was also okay and would not need surgery. Since the doctors had found nothing wrong, Pete checked out of the hospital. He returned to work on Monday. I returned to the prostate.

After a couple of months, the prostate became even more comfortable for me. Due to the swelling, I had more room than ever before. The prostate was now so large that it almost completely blocked off bowel movements. Pete went for another check-up. This time the doctor told Pete that he was in an emergency situation and had to go straight to the hospital for surgery. Pete complied and the doctor did a good job of correcting the problem. Later Pete was told there was no malignancy and he was released from the hospital. But the anesthetic used during surgery had weakened Pete's lungs. I moved back up there.

Pete's wheezing became worse over the next few months. I was having a good old time in my residence. Lots of room, lots of redness, and lots of mucus to float around on.

About this time, Pete was in a car accident. He was sitting in his car in traffic at a standstill when a car rear-ended him at about 55 miles per hour. Pete's car was shoved out of the traffic lane and up onto a median. The car had more than $3000 worth of damage, but Pete seemed unhurt except for a whiplash to his neck. More weakening.

Over the next few days, Pete's breathing deteriorated. He felt that he could barely get any oxygen in. He went back to the hospital for more tests. This time he was told he had asthma. He was given bronchodilators and Ventolin.

Pete went back to work. With the aid of medication, Pete could now breathe, but he was not getting better. He was still working a full schedule, but he lacked stamina and strength. He could no longer play racquetball in the mornings before work, nor could he do any strenuous work. All he could do was just get through the day.

Pete began to slow down. Pete's breathing was labored, and he often had pain after eating. He had frequent chest infections, copious mucus, and he could not speak above a whisper. He continued to work, but when he got home it would take him 15 minutes to climb the few stairs at the entrance of his home. Worst of all, Pete started noticing that food was going through him *whole*. His bowel movements were showing whole chunks of undigested food. In spite of the fact that he was eating three large meals a day, Pete's weight was dropping fast. Within three weeks Pete's shoulders became visibly thinner and the bones protruded.

Still the doctors couldn't find me, Al the Allergy. I'm so good at what I do. Mimicking is my specialty. Pete's doctor found nothing wrong except for the asthma.

It was a Sunday and Pete lay in bed late. He thought about his health problems. He was weak and tired. He knew he was slowly dying. He realized he had to change something quickly. He decided to call a friend who lived a thousand miles away. His friend was both a medical doctor and a doctor of naturopathy. Pete whispered his story of what had been happening to him over the last months.

His friend became alarmed when he heard the story. He recognized the symptoms of immune system failure. He wanted a blood sample sent immediately. In the meantime, he air-shipped an extract

4

of whole thymus to Pete. The thymus gland is the master gland of the immune system.

Pete was then tested by a local doctor of chiropractic who was proficient in allergic disorders. Pete was reacting to everything in his environment. He found out he was allergic to all except five foods. He was allergic to the carpets and drapes, any chemical with which he came into contact including perfume and hair sprays, and even the upholstery in his car. He was a universal reactor.

At first I wasn't worried. Even when I've been discovered for the allergy that I am, it rarely makes a difference. Antihistamines seldom bother me. They just make the person feel a little better while I'm still around snug as ever in the person's body.

Pete took action. He moved into the guest bedroom of his own house where there was no carpet and only a small curtain. He ate only the five foods allowed and took vitamin preparations to build his immune system. He took digestive enzymes so his food would digest. Then one day he made an important discovery. He found that when he accidentally ate something that he reacted to, and the intense pain started under his liver, he could take certain enzymes and the pain would go away within 20 minutes! Even the pain killers at the hospital couldn't do that!

Pete started to improve. His immune system was slowly getting stronger. Now I was worried. The immune system is the only thing that can boot me out of my comfortable home.

Pete was now out of pain, his blood pressure was returning to normal, his voice returned and his breathing improved. He was able to eat a few more foods. His energy was starting to return also. In a few weeks, Pete was feeling more vigorous. All his symptoms were gone except for the asthma. As long as he took the asthma medication he felt fairly normal.

Now I was really alarmed! I had lost all my residences in Pete's body except for the lungs and bronchi. At the rate Pete was going, it looked as though I might lose them as well. But then Pete made an error in judgment.

Pete was feeling so good and was so happy to have survived his ordeal that he became careless. He began to eat whatever he liked again, and didn't pay attention to his rest. His immune system had reached a plateau and it stayed there. While Pete did not seem to become any worse, he also did not continue to improve. With the medications there were only a few breathing symptoms, and the vitamin supplements and enzymes kept him from getting worse. It looks like Pete will stay this way for a while. And it looks like I, Al the Allergy, will have a home for just a little while longer.

# 2

# Recognizing Allergy and Its Causes

The greatest challenge with allergy is recognizing it. We have been conditioned to think of allergy as being limited to such symptoms as runny eyes, sniffling nose, sinus problems, skin rashes, asthma and hay fever. However, allergy is much more insidious and extensive. It can also take the form of arthritis, gall bladder disease, intractable headache, Crohn's disease, depression, psychotic behavior, and more than one hundred other conditions not normally thought of as allergy. Allergy does not cause *every* disease, but it can be involved in almost *any* disease. It can play an integral role in the development of disease. It is so prevalent that if you have not been told the cause of your health problems or symptoms, you should consider allergy first.

Allergy is not usually considered to be life-threatening – who ever died from a runny nose? This lack of understanding persists in spite of the fact that almost everyone has heard about anaphylaxis, a massive allergic reaction that kills in minutes. Few other diseases can kill so rapidly. Anaphylaxis kills within sixteen minutes to two hours after contact with an allergen, whether it is from a bee sting, a handful of peanuts or a penicillin shot.

The slow progress of most cases of allergy is even less understood. Over the course of months and years, allergy can so weaken the body systems that other life-threatening diseases gain a foothold in the body. This is because allergies, whether you recognize them or not, weaken the immune system over time so that the body cannot defend itself from foreign invaders and tissue degeneration. The most common way allergy kills is not by anaphylactic shock reaction, but by the slow, insidious, multiple-symptom syndrome.

How do you learn to recognize allergy? You can suspect allergy any time you have an inflammation anywhere in your body. Allergy follows the cardinal signs of inflammation: pain, swelling, heat and redness. Whenever you have allergy, one and usually more of these symptoms are present.

If the allergic reaction is near the skin, you will often see all four of these signs. For example, hives will produce the swelling, look red, feel warm, and be painful. Sometimes the reaction will occur internally where there are few nerve endings. In this case, the tissue may be swollen, red and hot, but you may not feel it because of the lack of nerve endings. Depending on where the reaction takes place, you will have different symptoms. Remember this little known fact: allergy can occur anywhere in the body, even in the brain.

Inflammation is designated by the word ending *itis*. If an allergic reaction which produces inflammation occurs in the sinuses, it is called sinusitis; in the bowel, colitis; in the joints, arthritis; in the bronchi, bronchitis; and in the skin, dermatitis.

## Causes of Allergy

What causes allergy? There are usually several causes. Allergy is the result of various insults to the body, coupled with a person's unique hereditary background and his individual metabolic state. Certain body patterns and metabolic states have been associated with the production of allergic symptoms. The fact that allergic disease is polycausal (has many causes), has led to medical confusion: doctors look for only one cause, then try to find a drug to offset the symptoms. Since no single cause can be found, allergic symptoms are often ignored or attributed to mental or emotional stress.

**Heredity:** A person inherits the *predisposition* to allergy, rather than the specific allergy. Therefore it is the *tendency* to become allergic to a foreign substance that is inherited. The greater the incidence of allergy in a family, the greater the tendency for the offspring to develop allergy. If one parent is allergic, the chances of the children being allergic are 50 to 58 percent. If both parents are allergic, the likelihood of the children being allergic is 67 to 100 percent.

Research confirms that a developing fetus in the uterus can demonstrate the hallmark of allergy, IgE antibody formation in the liver and lungs, by the eleventh week of gestation. IgE has also been found in the amniotic fluid (the fluid surrounding the fetus) at thirteen weeks. No IgE has been found in the arterial blood of the umbilical cord, leading doctors to believe that the placenta does not allow direct transfer of maternal blood containing IgE to the fetus. There are, however, studies that show that *allergens* transferred placentally can lead to intra-uterine sensitization. Allergies to penicillin, wheat, milk and eggs have been the most frequently documented.

**Biochemical Individuality:** A person's metabolic pattern or state is unique to that person. In some people the genetic requirements for nutrients can be much higher than "normal" to prevent disease. In others metabolic individuality can cause them to react very differently to various substances.

Allergy appears to increase with advancing age. As a person ages, he tends to have weakened resistance due to a weakened immune system, various stages of organ degeneration and having had more time to accumulate toxic substances which lead to metabolic overload. Also, nutritional deficiencies often increase as a person ages since they accumulate over time from the person's eating patterns.

Emotionally stressful situations can lead to diminished immune system function. Physical stress can increase nutrient requirements, leading to deficiency. Nutrient deficiency further stresses the immune system. Poor diet affects the body's ability to fight disease. It leaves the body unprotected. As one organ or body system loses its ability to function at peak performance, it affects other organs and systems. These other organs and systems must now do more work to compensate for the one that is stressed. As malnutrition continues, these accommodating organs and systems become stressed and lose their ability to function optimally. You cannot affect one part of the body without affecting other parts. According to James C. Breneman, MD, author of *Basics of Food Allergy,* food allergy and intolerance are technically forms of malnutrition.

**Toxic Load:** Frequency and extent of exposure plays a large role in allergy. Increasing exposure to a substance causes toxic load to build faster in the body. People are increasingly exposed to a variety of industrial pollutants, pesticides and chemicals. The air, food and water have all been altered in recent years leading to varying degrees of toxic load.

**Drugs:** The vast quantity of prescription and over-the-counter drugs available today is indeed astounding. Allergic reactions to drugs have been well documented, although the information has not been well distributed. The drug most often causing allergic reactions is penicillin. The second most allergic drug is aspirin. Drugs contribute directly to allergy by decreasing liver function, increasing chemical overload and destroying enzyme systems. Other drugs frequently associated with allergic reactions include:

| | |
|---|---|
| sulfonamides | sedative-hypnotics (barbiturates) |
| anti tuberculosis drugs | antimalarial drugs |
| anti convulsants | antipsychotic tranquilizers |
| blood pressure drugs | antiserum and vaccines |
| heavy metals (including gold) | antiarrhythmics (heart agents) |

**Infant Formula:** Feeding infant formula to babies increases the frequency of allergy. Dr. Breneman states: "The highest incidence of lifetime milk allergy is found in this iatrogenically conditioned group." Iatrogenic means doctor-caused, presumably by prescribing cow's milk infant formula.

**Illness:** After infectious illness changes can take place in the body that allow allergy to emerge. The body will react more readily to allergic stimuli. For example, asthma may occur after a bout with measles or pneumonia. Infection of the intestine can make its lining more permeable to undigested food particles, producing allergic symptoms. Biochemical changes take place in the body during prolonged illness, leading to decreased resistance to allergic stimuli. Toxins produced by the yeast *Candida albicans* play a major part in allergy. These toxins include acetaldehyde, carbon monoxide, alcohol, steroid substances and up to one hundred other substances not completely identified. The more frequent the exposure the greater the incidence of allergy.

Dr. Theron G. Randolph, a pioneer in clinical ecology, found that a person may acquire or lose sensitivities depending on how often they are exposed to a given food or substance. Dr. Randolph estimates that for every one allergy that we recognize at least two more remain hidden.

**Stress:** Stress in any form, whether it is emotional, chemical, or environmental can contribute to allergic symptoms. Any stress that is beyond a person's ability to cope leads to adaptive changes physically and mentally. However, much "mental stress" has now been identified as being due to chemicals in the environment, Candida infections, toxins in food and electromagnetic disharmonies previously unperceived by the individual.

**Dental Fillings:** Mercury is a component of the silver amalgam used in dental fillings. Mercury is highly toxic to the nerves and immune system. This toxicity has historically been illustrated by the "mad hatter" syndrome, whereby hat makers became mentally ill after using mercury in the production of hats. Mercury in fillings of the teeth leeches out over the years. It also produces toxic mercury vapor in the mouth. Bacteria and fungi found in the mouth are capable of converting mercury into an even more toxic product called methyl mercury. Mercury is one of many toxins capable of contributing to chemical overload in the body, blocking enzymes and leading to degenerative diseases, including allergies.

**Foods:** Repeated consumption of a specific food plays a part in allergy by depleting enzyme systems. Most people eat only a very few foods – the ones they like best. For the majority of people, this is approximately fifteen foods, but they eat them in a variety of ways. If a person particularly likes potatoes, he will eat them frequently as baked potatoes, french fries, hash browns or potato chips. Beef may be steak, hamburger or stew. Daily overeating of a few specific foods has the effect of stressing the enzyme systems to handle that food. If the food is also an allergenic food, the body's capacity to deal with it is greatly diminished. Food is man's primary potential allergen and addictant. This is because everybody eats every day. As a result of the quantity eaten, food provides the greatest consistent stimulation to the body.

An article by Hugh A. Sampson, MD, which appeared in the *Journal of the American College of Nutrition* (Volume 9, Number 4, 1990), states, "The development of food allergy is the result of an interaction between food allergens, the gastrointestinal tract and the immune system."

Albert H. Rowe, MD, a pioneer on the subject of food allergy, has shown that food allergy can be responsible for any symptom in any system of the body and it can manifest itself at any age.

**Everybody breathes:** In some people, pollens, dust spores, insect debris, animal danders and airborne chemicals play a major role in allergy. Not everybody uses tobacco, alcohol and drugs. However, when these substances are used, the body can be stressed even more and at an earlier age.

## Understanding Allergy

The words *allergic to* imply that the allergenic substance is the cause. In fact, this only demonstrates that the person, for one reason or another, has lost the normal ability to cope appropriately with that substance. The substance itself is not the cause, it is only the *trigger* of the allergic reaction.

Many allergic symptoms are characteristically ignored. No one disputes that classic symptoms such as runny nose, watery eyes and skin rashes are allergic conditions. No one disputes that allergy is involved when a person bites into a peanut butter cookie and dies of anaphylactic shock. It is amazing that if allergy can produce symptoms as mild as a runny nose or as life-threatening as anaphylactic shock, that the range of symptoms between these two extremes is seldom recognized. Why are these intermediary symptoms rarely linked to allergy?

The whole field of allergy is vastly under-explored. We know more about the Arctic Circle and the migration of whales than we do about allergy. Compounding the situation, much of what we do know about allergy, and what has been recently discovered is not generally known to the public, but is tucked away on the shelves of medical libraries.

The truth is that any symptom which your body is capable of producing can be of allergic origin. Not every symptom is allergy, but any symptom can be allergy. What about ulcers, high blood pressure, gall bladder disease, bed-wetting, arthritis or enlarged prostate? New information is showing that these conditions can be of allergic origin. We now have volumes of reports from all over the world indicating that allergy can involve any part of the body.

There are almost as many definitions of allergy as there are authors. Some books on allergy never offer a definition without getting into complicated discussions of the immune system involving antigens, antibodies, leukocytes, etc. There is a reason for these differences among authors. To understand the differences, it is necessary to look into the history of allergy.

# 3

# Old Dogma Hinders Healing

*A*llergy is not new. The symptoms of allergy have been described since ancient times. The death in 2641 BC of King Menes, an Egyptian pharaoh, after being stung by a bee, sounds very much like what we describe as anaphylactic shock. The Babylonian Talmud offered advice on building up tolerance to eggs in persons who experienced distress after eating them. The famous saying, "One man's meat is another man's poison," dates from Lucretius about two thousand years ago.

Around 1906, things started to change. The term *allergy* was coined from two Greek words meaning altered reactivity. It meant that an allergy was an adverse response to a substance by one person but not by most people. For example, pollen could give some people symptoms such as runny nose and eyes, but others experienced no reaction. Around the same time Frances Hare, an Australian physician, wrote two volumes titled *The Food Factor in Disease*. These volumes detail cases in which many common symptoms including mental symptoms are linked to eating common foods.

For the next twenty years doctors documented reactions to specific food allergens. However, the vast array of symptoms coupled with the vast array of causative agents including food, chemicals and inhalants presented problems from a scientific standpoint. How do you study a substance that seemingly causes headaches in one person, rashes in another and depression in yet another, particularly when the same substance causes no demonstrable symptoms in most people?

In 1926, a milestone decision was made. In that year, European allergists met with American allergists and agreed to limit the definition of allergy to immunological types of reactions only. Reactions involving the immune system produce antibodies in the tissues. Here was physical evidence that could be categorized and measured. Before 1926, allergy was considered to be any altered reaction to a common substance. After 1926, allergies were allergen-antibody reactions involving the immune system only. This decision was reinforced around 1967 when the immunoglobulin IgE was discovered. IgE was the first recognized antibody involved in immune-type allergic reactions.

This historic decision of 1926 is of profound importance to you today if you suffer from allergies. It means that if you go to a traditional or orthodox allergist for testing, he will diagnose only reactions involving IgE antibody production as being allergy. Any other reactions and symptoms that you may be experiencing are likely to be ignored. Food sensitivities often do not produce immunological reactions from skin testing, although they may produce a wide variety of symptoms throughout the body. Therefore, they may not be considered to be allergies. Many doctors estimate that up to two-thirds of allergic-like reactions may be in this category.

Following the 1926 decision, two groups of allergists appeared. The "scientific," orthodox allergists, who worked primarily with molds, dusts, grasses and pollens, required an allergen-antibody reaction as a basis for diagnosis. The other group was considered unorthodox. This group continued to study foods and other substances even though an immunological reaction could not necessarily be found. Research grants from major food manufacturers went mostly to the orthodox groups. Little money was available for the doctors who continued to study foods.

In 1965, Dr. Randolph Moss, along with other doctors, founded the Society for Clinical Ecology. These doctors recognized the ecological aspects, including the effects of foods, in many medical problems. Unfortunately, clinical ecology is not taught in medical school. Doctors learn about it through postgraduate courses, private reading and clinical observations.

## Terminology

Because of controversy in the medical establishment, many terms have been devised by doctors to describe various adverse reactions. The terms *hypersensitivity, intolerance, idiosyncrasy, maladaptive, allergic-like, atopic* and others have been used to describe the various abnormal reactions occurring in the body after contact with an environmental stimulus.

In the strictest sense of the word, *hypersensitivity* is an adverse food reaction occurring as a result of an abnormal immunological response, while the term *intolerance* is considered to be the result of a non-immunologic response of the body. It is fairly well agreed that food intolerance is responsible for the majority of adverse reactions to food. Many doctors believe that intolerance results not so much from the food, but rather from things that are in the food such as additives or naturally occurring toxins, or even from a metabolic disorder of the person involved.

Proof is difficult to establish. Most laboratory blood tests deal primarily in identifying the IgE antibody and fail to screen for reactions that may produce the IgG, IgA or IgM antibodies. The most accepted diagnostic test for allergy, the elimination diet and subsequent reintroduction of suspected substances, does not differentiate between the two terms, *allergy* and *intolerance.*

In addition, the term *antigen* designates a molecule that is recognized by the immune system and induces an immune response with the production of antibodies such as IgG, IgM and IgA or T-cells. An *allergen i*s an antigen that induces an IgE mediated response.

The *Atlas of Allergies* by Philip Fireman, MD and Raymond G. Slavin, MD states, "This immunologic definition of allergy is accepted by almost all but not every allergist since non-immune processes can influence the pathogenesis of allergic diseases with recognized immune etiologies."

With disagreement in the medical community and the confusing variety of possible terms involved in allergy, a simplified definition will be used throughout this book. The term *allergy* will be used to describe any heightened or exaggerated reaction which develops after more than one exposure to a common substance and which does not affect the majority of people. The term *allergen* will be used to describe the initiating substance of the reaction.

## The Vital Choice: Relief or Wellness?

There are many products on the market promising to relieve, control, manage or attack allergy. These products work by interfering with various chemical reactions that normally occur in the body. An example is antihistamines. These drugs may relieve symptoms by preventing histamine from being released from certain cells in the body. While antihistamines are the most common drugs used to treat allergic symptoms, they are not without side effects. A major side effect is drowsiness. If this occurs, driving a motor vehicle or operating machinery is not recommended. Another common side effect is dryness of the mouth, nose and throat. Blurred vision, dizziness, loss of appetite, nausea, upset stomach, low blood pressure, headache and loss of coordination are less common side effects. Antihistamines sometimes cause nervousness, restlessness or insomnia. Many over-the-counter products sold for allergies contain amphetamine-like nasal decongestants. Adverse reactions to these products include jitteriness, sleeplessness and potential heart problems. At any rate, relief or control of symptoms is all that is offered.

There is a difference between relieving or controlling a symptom and actually getting well, whereby health returns. Using drugs against allergy cannot get you well. It *is* possible to get well from allergies *without* drugs. By understanding what allergy is and how it works in the body, a person can free himself from allergy using alternate, healthful methods.

By using the innovative approach explained in this book, it is possible to recover from allergies without having to get rid of the family pet, without moving to another location, without allergy shots, without rotating foods and keeping diet diaries and without cooking allergy-free recipes for the rest of your life.

Getting well from allergy is more than just relieving, controlling and managing symptoms. It means that health returns and you no longer have a condition that you must keep treating. While there are those who will tell you this is not possible, hundreds of other people have already recovered from allergy and lead an allergy-free life. The only way you can be sure is to investigate the matter for yourself. Then make a decision as to the course of action that you are going to take. This should be an informed decision based on facts, not prejudice.

Dr. William Philpott makes the following statement: "We must always keep in mind that the greatest enemy of any science, or any discovery of truth, is a closed mind. Accordingly, we should continue to seek the courage to ask impertinent questions which will shake out complacency and challenge our minds to look deeper into the great mystery of the human body."

# 4

# New Ideas about Allergy

The new, broader understanding of allergy is based on five essential concepts.

## Concept One:
### *The body tends to homeostasis.*
Homeostasis is defined as a tendency to uniformity or stability in the normal body state. In a healthy body all organs and tissues of the body perform functions that help maintain conditions of equilibrium.

It sounds like a tall order, considering all of the millions of activities that take place in your body each day. For example, all of the blood in the circulatory system flows through your body an average of once a minute when your body is at rest. It circulates about six times a minute during exercise. In your body, seven to ten million new cells are formed every second. At the same time the blood is carrying oxygen and nutrients to all of the estimated 70 to 100 trillion cells in your body. Your body has the wisdom to handle all of this without your conscious help.

If nothing intervenes, the body will remain running perfectly. If trauma or other irritation occurs to the body, it will make the necessary corrections to return to a state of homeostasis. If the traumatic irritation is prolonged, the body will still strive to make corrections. However, when the stress is of such long duration that the body is unable to make corrections, it will compensate by calling in other systems or substituting other materials for the job. Eventually some of these compensating systems become exhausted. The body then cannot return to homeostasis and remains out of balance. This is like a gyroscope starting to wind down: it simply cannot run smoothly and efficiently anymore and starts to wobble.

The primary sources of prolonged trauma and irritation to the body are habits, lifestyle and beliefs. For example, drinking alcohol every day is a source of irritation for the body. The body tries to compensate for the loss of minerals, the lack of oxygen and the toxicity to the liver. If the stress continues long enough, the body will go out of balance and call in compensatory mechanisms in order to survive. Regular over-consumption of alcohol is an example of a habit affecting homeostasis.

For every action in the body, there is also an opposite action. You have muscles to open your hand and other muscles to close your hand. You have hormones to speed up metabolism and hormones to slow it down. The body stays in balance by constantly making adjustments day and night, day after day and year after year. It's sort of like staying in the middle of a teeter-totter. Then along comes a lifestyle that pushes you out to one end. Eventually, the exhausted body cannot make its way back to the middle. Symptoms appear. The body is telling you that it is not in homeostasis and a correction should be made allowing the body to move back toward health. If this is not done, that symptom will eventually turn into something more serious.

Eczema in the infant often becomes asthma in the adult. Low blood sugar often becomes adult onset diabetes. When an allergic symptom appears, the body is saying that it is struggling to cope with its environment, both internal and external. It is imperative to change something now to take stress off the body. A body that is in homeostasis cannot be exhibiting allergy. It will not react abnormally to any substance. A body in homeostasis does not have any symptoms. It has only health.

## Concept Two:
### *Any symptom can be allergy.*

Any symptom or condition of the body, anywhere in the body, at any time, can be allergy, particularly when that symptom is not explainable in other terms. Food allergies in particular are poorly understood. When you eat a banana and get an immediate pain in your abdomen or stomach, you realize that there is a connection between eating the banana and getting the pain. But if the only response to that banana comes days later in the form of a swollen joint, you do not necessarily recognize that there is a relationship between what you ate and the response that occurred. Much "masked" or "delayed" allergy falls into this category.

Allergy is considered an altered reaction – the reaction that one person will get to a substance that does not affect other people. Anything a person puts in his mouth is capable of eliciting an allergic response, even tap water. It's not the water itself but what is in the water, such as chlorine, fluoride and up to one hundred other chemicals, that can precipitate the reaction. When tap water is consumed, chemicals enter the body, but only some individuals will get an allergic response. A person can also have an allergic response to the air that he breathes. This is, of course, more readily understood, because we have a greater awareness of the toxicity of tobacco smoke and city smog and the effects of pollen.

Doctors who have worked extensively with allergy, and especially with food allergy, are astounded over the wide range of symptoms that can be observed in patients. It is an extraordinary concept that PMS, epilepsy, bloody diarrhea, backache and swollen arthritic joints can be produced by common everyday foods. The idea that foods, considered nourishment for the body, are capable of producing a major illness may be difficult to comprehend.

Milk is the most common allergen. The patient who drinks lots of milk is aghast when it turns out to be a cause of his colitis. This patient may have believed that he was doing "something good" for himself. A person who drinks "tons" of milk often turns out to be calcium deficient. How can this possibly be, he wonders? If you react allergically to a food, it is difficult for the body to absorb its nutrients.

Dr. James C. Breneman writes, "The incidence of diet-related problems is greater than the incidence of any other type of illness affecting mankind." He estimates that 60 percent of the population has unknown food allergies or intolerances. Other authors estimate the figure to be closer to 80 percent. It is important that people increase their awareness of the scope of allergy as a possible cause of their symptoms. Most people do not think of gall bladder symptoms as being caused by allergy, especially if they have never had classic allergic symptoms such as hay fever or skin rashes. Many people have little awareness that bed-wetting in a child can be allergy, especially to milk. This is particularly true when the child does not appear to have any other allergic symptoms. One lady said recently that she did not have allergies. All she had was arthritis. She did not realize that allergy often plays a role in this disease. If you have allergic symptoms that are not the traditional type, you will often be told there is nothing wrong with you, or that it is "all in your mind."

Doctors have limited awareness and knowledge in the area of food allergy because:

1. Food allergy is not taught at medical schools.
2. Doctors must get training in food allergy from post-graduate seminars or from clinical experience.
3. Many doctors consider food allergy to be fantasy.
4. Orthodox allergists recognize only immunological-type reactions. They do not consider anything else to be allergy, even in the face of obvious clinical symptoms.

If the scope of allergy has not been taught to doctors, how are they to recognize it? The fact is that most allergy goes untreated and unrecognized while the patient must put up with chronic debilitating symptoms.

## Concept Three:
### *Symptoms appear when allergic load is reached.*

In the book *Clinical Ecology*, Dr. Lawrence Dickey states, "It would be surprising if people were not allergic to pesticides put into the ground and sprayed on crops, to flour 'improvers,' anti-staling agents, emulsifying compounds, artificial colorings, preservatives and the whole terrifying array of potentially toxic substances now being added to our food in order to improve appearance, flavor, shelf-life and profitability."

It has been estimated that more than five pounds of these toxic materials are taken into each person's body each year. The combined and accumulated effects are not known, but we are seeing an increase of observable abnormal reactions in the body. Because the immune system is programmed to defend us from foreign substances, allergy or intolerance is one of the body's initial responses. After many years of being in a hyper-excited state, the immune system becomes exhausted. This leaves the body with lowered defenses, which can later lead to many forms of chronic degenerative disease.

It is not known whether the human body has built sufficient enzyme systems to eliminate or neutralize all the toxic effects of the smorgasbord of chemicals taken in. It is known that oxidative enzymes and certain vitamins and minerals are necessary to eliminate or neutralize the toxins. However, with more than five pounds of these chemicals going into the body each year, year after year, the question remains whether we are over-taxing our body's ability to produce the substances necessary to eliminate the chemicals. As the nutrient value of our food goes down and the chemical content rises, can our bodies meet the demand? When the demand is greater than the supply, the body must pull in compensatory mechanisms in order to defend itself. This is like running out of money and trying to use your garden hose to buy your food. It doesn't work as well as money and you soon run out of garden hoses as well.

Allergic load is the amount of chemicals, food allergens and inhalant pollutants that a person can be exposed to before symptoms appear. It is the sum total of toxicity (toxic load) accumulated before systems in the body malfunction, producing symptoms and alerting you to the fact that something is wrong.

Allergic or toxic load is different for everyone. People are born with varying genetic strengths and weaknesses. The child of an alcoholic mother has a much smaller health reserve to start with than the child of a healthy mother. Toxic load also depends upon *what* you are exposed to. Before it was known how toxic asbestos is, workers in an asbestos factory built up a toxic load of asbestos in their lungs faster than people of the general population.

When a certain point of toxicity is reached in the body from any source, whether it was ingested, inhaled, injected or absorbed through the skin, allergy is one of the first symptoms to appear. Whether the allergy is recognized or not depends on the experience of the doctor who is consulted. Many doctors do not yet realize that ulcers or gastritis can be allergic symptoms. The body will tolerate insults only to a certain level before it reacts and symptoms appear. It is similar to a mother tolerating the annoying loud noise her child makes for a time before she explodes with anger. The body is saying, "Hey, I've reached my limit. Beyond this point sickness will result. Change something now."

That swollen joint, headache or gastritis is a sign telling you something is wrong. If you ignore the sign and proceed full speed ahead, you can expect increasingly severe symptoms.

In the book *The McDougall Plan,* Dr. John A. McDougall states, "The body's immune system has a limited capacity to deal with allergens and when the system becomes overloaded, allergic symptoms appear. If you can reduce the intake of allergens from one source, such as food, you will ease the burden of the entire immune system. In this way you can help your body deal with other sources of allergies, such as particles in the air."

Each person's ability to metabolize toxins, pollens, foods and chemicals can differ considerably according to his own biochemical makeup. But consider that almost every food available in a modern supermarket has been tampered with in some way to the detriment of its nutritional and enzyme content. Unless it is certified organically-grown, all fresh produce has been sprayed, has been grown on mineral-deficient soil and has absorbed constituents of artificial fertilizers which may contain herbicides. Some produce has been irradiated, which destroys its enzyme content. Boxed foods are all enzyme deficient as they are processed at high temperatures and they may also contain chemical additives. Frozen foods may be blanched or cooked and often contain salt, sugar and chemical additives. Canned foods are subjected to very high temperatures, destroying their enzymes and some nutrients. All this contributes toward the individual's toxic load, regardless of his resistance level.

## Concept Four:
### *Allergy has no single cause.*

For many diseases, there is no such thing as "the cause." We are told through the media that "they" are looking for "the cause" of cancer and "the cause" of arthritis. Why is it assumed that there is only one cause? The truth is that in chronic conditions, there isn't. That there is only one cause for each disease is an assumption that will eventually be proven wrong for many degenerative conditions.

The problem is that the one cause-one disease model is the only one that fits current scientific testing criteria. Robert C. Atkins, MD, in his book *Dr. Atkins' Health Revolution,* explains that the double blind study is the criterion scientists use. "The double blind is an excellent test for evaluating pharmaceutical and single variables. I agree that, when it is applicable, it should be used. The problem is that, as the protocols get stricter in their exclusion of subjectivity, the area of applicability becomes narrower and narrower. The real blind spot in the double blind is that the leadership in medicine continues to insist upon it as the only acceptable proof even though its applicability is so limited. The problem is that for many good therapies, a double-blind protocol cannot even be devised. "

A good example of this problem is provided by nutrients such as vitamins or minerals which are never found alone in nature. A nutrient may not test well as a single entity because it needs synergistic nutrients which work together to enhance its action. As a single nutrient, a vitamin may produce a weak effect. For example, vitamin C as ascorbic acid (a single nutrient) may be required in higher doses, but when used in conjunction with bioflavonoids will produce a better result with a lower dose.

As explained in Chapter two, allergy is the cumulative effect of many insults to the body which, over time, have overwhelmed the body's protective mechanisms. While dust may appear to be "the cause" of your runny nose, in reality it is only the trigger that activates the symptoms in an already compromised organism.

## Concept Five:
*Taking personal responsibility leads to wellness.*

Most people truly want to be healthy but have only a vague idea of what to do to achieve health. Much of their information on health has come from television and magazine articles. As a result, they may be proud of the fact that they are taking antacids to get calcium, taking aspirin to avoid heart attacks and switching from butter to margarine to lower their cholesterol. All of these unhealthy practices contribute to illness. To be healthy, you must do healthy things. The problem is that people do not know or are not sure about what these healthy things are.

There are actually six things the body requires to stay healthy. In order to build health, the body requires food, water, air, sunshine, exercise and sleep. Most of these are well understood by the average person. People usually have a very realistic idea of the amount of sleep they require. They know that exercise and fresh air are necessary and that moderate exposure to sunshine is healthful. People also agree that water is required each day and that it should be pure and clean. The big hang-up is about food. Here, people are very, very unsure of what foods are good for them and why. Much of their knowledge about food is based on beliefs, not facts. The information contained in this book will not only provide facts on which foods are healthful, but also a new understanding of why some foods are healthful and others are not.

Health is your responsibility. Remember the old saying "You can lead a horse to water but you can't make him drink"? It's the same with health. You can be shown the path to better health, but only you can follow the path. You can learn what foods to eat, but only you can eat them. In the movie *The Wizard of Oz,* Dorothy was led down the yellow brick road, but in the end only she could get herself home. She had placed all her hopes of getting home on the power of the wizard, but after she discovered the wizard was a fake, she found that the power to get herself home was within herself all the time.

It is the same way with health. The power to be healthy is within you at this very moment. The body is self-healing. All you need to do is discover how to tap into that power to obtain health. It is up to

28

you to learn what it is that your body needs. Your medical doctor looks only for a disease. The tests are there to diagnose or eliminate the possibility of disease. Tests are not done to determine your individual biochemical requirements to stay healthy. Your body will stay healthy as long as you give it what it needs and do not interfere with it, either knowingly or unknowingly. That could mean changing your lifestyle, diet or beliefs. It is your responsibility to make those changes if you wish to be healthy. Disease, including allergy, is the result of a lifetime of destructive habits. If you don't like the result, you must change the input. Health cannot be forced on anyone. However, anyone wanting to be healthy can make the changes required to accomplish that goal.

# 5

# The Secret Life of an Allergen

Many types of allergic reactions have been documented. Understanding how these reactions occur and how they affect the tissues of the body gives clues not only to recognizing them but also to eliminating them.

Our encounter with an allergen begins with the immune system – the primary defense system of the body. It is made up of various tissues, glands and organs, such as the thymus gland, spleen, tonsils, lymph nodes and bone marrow. White blood cells, called lymphocytes, are major defenders. Billions of lymphocytes patrol the blood stream looking for and destroying invading viruses, bacteria, parasites and other foreign substances.

Allergy affects the immune system in a number of ways. It affects it directly when an antibody, a product of the immune system, reacts immediately and specifically with the allergen. It can also affect the immune system indirectly. If the adverse reaction initially takes place outside the immune system, the immune system is eventually called in to "clean up" the result of the reaction. Either way the immune system is involved sooner or later. In this sense all allergic reactions are immunological, even if they do not fall within the allergists' rather narrow definition which requires that an antibody be demonstrably present. All allergy puts stress on the immune system.

Normal body cells are coated with a special protective protein that the immune system can recognize. Because of this protective coat, normal cells are not attacked by the immune system. Dead tissues and foreign particles have no protective coat, and are phagocytized (eaten) by cells of the immune system.

A person can become sensitized when a foreign substance enters the body by any means. It could happen by inhalation, ingestion, injection or absorption through the skin. When a person is exposed to this foreign substance, antibodies are built by plasma cells of the immune system. When the substance or allergen is taken in again, it reacts with the specified antibodies. When the allergen contacts an antibody, an immediate reaction takes place producing symptoms, usually within minutes or hours.

If the allergen reacts with lymphocytes, a delayed form of allergy occurs hours or even days later. This delayed form is not nearly so well recognized by professionals. For example, if you eat strawberries and hives appear within hours, you will probably realize that strawberries were a precipitating factor. But if the symptoms appear two to three days later you often will have forgotten by then that you ate strawberries and you are less likely to link the two events together.

Allergic reaction runs one of two courses: symptoms can appear and subsequently disappear, or they can produce permanent pathological changes.

## The Classic (IgE) Allergic Reaction

Classic cases of allergic reaction involve antibodies. Antibodies are gamma globulins called immunoglobulins. IgE antibodies are synthesized by plasma cells located primarily under the mucosal surfaces of the respiratory and digestive tract. Antibodies make up about 20 percent of the plasma proteins of the body. There are five major types: IgE, IgG, IgM, IgA and IgD. Seventy-five percent of the antibodies in a normal person are of the IgG type.

IgE makes up only a small proportion, about one percent, but it is particularly involved in allergy. It is the IgE antibody that the allergist looks for when diagnosing allergy. After the IgE antibody is formed, it becomes bound to receptor sites on white blood cells known as mast cells and basophils. A single blood basophil can have up to

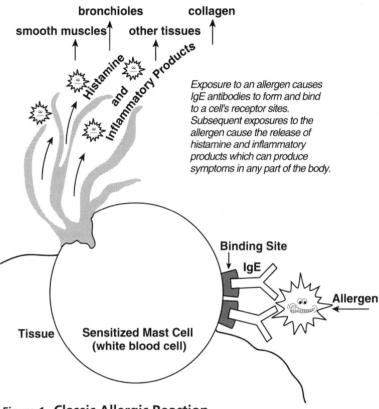

bronchioles   collagen
smooth muscles   other tissues

Histamine and Inflammatory Products

Exposure to an allergen causes IgE antibodies to form and bind to a cell's receptor sites. Subsequent exposures to the allergen cause the release of histamine and inflammatory products which can produce symptoms in any part of the body.

Binding Site
IgE
Allergen
Tissue   Sensitized Mast Cell (white blood cell)

*Figure 1.* **Classic Allergic Reaction**

100,000 IgE receptor sites. A non-allergic person will have only 20 to 50 percent of the receptors bound by antibodies. But nearly 100 percent of the sites will be occupied by IgE in an allergic individual.

Once IgE is bound to these sites the cells are considered to be sensitized. When the specific allergen is introduced again, a cascade of biochemical reactions takes place. This is the classic allergic reaction. The mast cells and basophils release potent chemicals into the tissues. The tissues most commonly affected are the smooth muscles of blood vessels, bronchioles and collagen or connective tissues. How-

33

ever, any tissue of the body can be affected. Antibodies can be formed in the blood stream and circulate. They attach to cells at other sites in the body. When re-exposed to the specific allergen, the allergic reaction takes place in what is now known as the "shock tissue."

## IgG

IgG immunoglobulins make up three-fourths of the antibodies of the blood stream. They are produced by white blood cells known as B-lymphocytes. IgG can attack and destroy most bacteria. Some researchers believe that IgG is involved in up to two-thirds of all allergic reactions.

IgG plays an important role in activating the complement system. Complement is a collective term used to describe about twenty different proteins, many of which are enzyme precursors. When IgG attaches to an invader or allergen, the complement system moves in. Through a series of chemical reactions in which the cell wall of the invader is "eaten" by the complement system enzymes, the invader ruptures and dies.

## IgA

It has been more recently discovered that the immunoglobulin IgA plays a major role in protection against allergy. Secretory IgA antibodies are found in saliva, tears, the blood stream and especially along the lining of the digestive tract. IgA's major role is to defend against foreign substances before they can enter the body.

Since the digestive system is often the first to contact an allergen, this is the place where significant allergic reactions occur. If an allergen is able to get past the IgA and enter the blood stream, it can be an indication of a *deficiency* of the secretory IgA that lines the digestive tract. This is why IgA can be considered a front line defender against allergens. Secretory IgA binds the allergens so that these compounds can be neutralized.

Statistics indicate that almost one-half of Americans are lacking secretory IgA. This means that allergens can penetrate the intestinal membranes unopposed and reach the blood stream. In addition, when an allergic food is eaten, some amount of secretory IgA is used up. If allergic food is eaten on a regular basis, this can contribute to secretory IgA deficiency.

In non-allergenic people, 3,000 to 5,000 milligrams of secretory IgA are produced daily. Allergic persons secrete substantially less secretory IgA than normal, and some persons secrete close to none at all. Some drugs which can contribute to secretory IgA deficiency are:

| | | |
|---|---|---|
| Aspirin | cortisone | Tagamet |
| Clinoril | Indocin | antibiotics |
| Naprosyn | antacids | birth control pill |

## Products of Allergic Reactions

Several substances are released during the various kinds of allergic reactions, causing far-reaching effects on tissue. These substances are described below:

**Histamine** is the best known substance released by the affected cells. It quickly spreads into the surrounding tissue. It acts directly on the small blood vessels making them "leaky" to the fluid of the body. This in turn leads to edema (swelling of the tissue), which then acts on nerve endings causing pain.

**Kinins:** Few doctors recognize kinin reactions as a source of intense pain. Kinins are a group of chemicals released into tissues as a result of inflammation. Of these, bradykinin is the most important. Bradykinin is one of the most potent vasodilators (dilators of blood vessels) known. It is about ten times more active than histamine or serotonin. It may be involved in up to two-thirds of allergic reactions. Bradykinin causes intense pain, as it is a very powerful stimulator of pain receptors. It also contracts smooth muscle, increases vascular permeability and dilates peripheral arterioles.

**Other Substances:** Other powerful substances that play a role in allergic disorders are leukotrienes, prostaglandins and thromboxins. Leukotrienes are highly inflammatory and can cause smooth muscle contraction. Prostaglandins are chemical substances that have been identified more recently. When activated, these hormones can cause powerful inflammation. Prostaglandins exist in almost every tissue of the body. They can have both vaso-constricting and vaso-dilating effects.

**Common thread:** What do all these substances have in common? They are all vasoactive, causing blood vessels to dilate or contract, and they are inflammatory, causing swelling, heat and pain. The dilation of local blood vessels causes loss of fluid into the tissue. Along with this fluid come increased numbers of proteins. The proteins tend to cluster in the tissues. These clusters are difficult for the lymphatics to absorb, so the proteins tend to pool there. The proteins pull water out of the circulation causing swelling. These clustered proteins attract excess sodium, which attracts still more fluid. Excess fluid and excess sodium create a lack of oxygen supply to the cells. This causes even more cell injury because cells need oxygen to survive. Decreased oxygen slows down cell function and causes acid to accumulate in the cell. It is believed that ischemic (lacking in blood) tissues also release toxins such as histamine, serotonin and tissue enzymes. Eventually the cells die.

## Immune Complexes

A common consequence of allergic reaction is the binding together of allergens and antibodies to form large allergen-antibody (immune) complexes. When formed, these immune complexes are deposited in tissues such as the kidneys, lungs, small blood vessels, liver and uterus. They can also be deposited in the arteries of the brain (eg. migraine sufferers) and in the brain membranes. Immune complexes release substances that activate a cascade of biochemical reactions. Additionally, complexes are capable of at least temporarily clogging up joints and blood vessels, resulting in local tissue injury. They can damage the filtering organs of the body, such as the kidneys and lymphatics. Immune complexes are responsible for up to 90 percent of kidney disease in humans. An increase in the permeability of the small blood vessels is required for these large immune complexes to be deposited in the various tissues. Histamine paves the way by causing leakiness of the capillaries.

## Anaphylaxis

The most life-threatening and dramatic of all allergic reactions is anaphylaxis. It occurs so rapidly that often therapy cannot be applied before death occurs. Anaphylaxis involves the whole body, causing similar shock symptoms to those one might see in a car accident victim. Symptoms begin within minutes of exposure to the allergen. Since the symptoms involve the whole body, the reaction is immediate and explosive. The victim may experience in rapid succession: a constricted feeling in the chest, dizziness, wheezing, nausea, vomiting or diarrhea, weakness, hoarseness, abdominal pain, skin manifestations, swelling and cyanosis (turning blue). Blood pressure can fall rapidly, and unconsciousness and death follows.

The number one cause of anaphylaxis is drugs, especially injected drugs. Injecting a substance bypasses the normal defense system of the body. Penicillin is the most common drug involved in anaphylaxis, with aspirin running a close second. Dyes used in X-ray diagnosis have also caused anaphylaxis, as have some anesthetics used in surgery. Peanuts and other nuts, eggs, fish and shellfish are the most common foods involved in anaphylaxis. Sulfites added to fruits, vegetables and processed foods are another frequent cause. Less common, but every bit as important, are the stinging insects. Insects such as bees and wasps cause deaths every year by anaphylaxis.

## Chronic Immune Suppression

Allergic reactions have a boomerang effect on the immune system. Although the immune system initially responds with a heightened reaction when an allergen is contacted, the white blood cell population then becomes depressed and remains lower than normal for as long as the exposure continues. This can cause chronic suppression of the immune system if the allergen is consumed or contacted on a daily basis.

# 6

# Symptoms of Allergy

Over one hundred symptoms have been medically recognized as being caused by allergic reactions to foods and environmental chemicals. No part of the body is immune to allergy. Listed below are the most common medically recognized symptoms.

**Neurological Symptoms:**

headache
depression
fatigue
sleeplessness (insomnia)
neuralgia
feeling of indecision
moodiness
melancholy (sad feelings)
withdrawal
apathy
emotional instability
impaired coordination
impaired comprehension
nervousness
stammering
fainting

aphasia (inability to speak
 or find the appropriate word)
mental lapses
blackouts
paranoid thinking
delusions
hallucinations
amnesia
coma
lethargy
disorientation
irritability
epilepsy
dizziness
violent behavior
hyperactivity

## Joint Symptoms:
arthritis                     arthralgia (joint pain)
swollen ankles

## Circulatory Symptoms:
chest pain                    irregular pulse
irregular heartbeat           anemia
hypertension                  edema
  (high blood pressure)       angina pectoris (heart pain)
hypotension                   phlebitis (inflammation
  (low blood pressure)          of a vein)

## Respiratory Symptoms:
runny nose                    coughing
asthma                        bronchitis
wheezing, shortness of breath sinusitis

## Gastrointestinal Symptoms:
excessive gas                 belching
diarrhea                      heartburn
constipation                  salivation
colitis                       food cravings
stomach cramps                gagging
nausea                        hunger pains
vomiting                      diverticulitis
abdominal pain                indigestion
canker sores                  hemorrhoids
peptic ulcers                 duodenal ulcer
gall bladder pain             bloating

## Skin Symptoms:
itching                       hives
eczema                        sweating
clammy skin                   acne
tendency towards              cracked skin
  bleeding and bruising

**Musculo-skeletal Symptoms:**

neckache                          backache
myalgia (muscle pain)

**Hormonal Symptoms:**

dysmenorrhea                      impotence
frigidity

**Other Symptoms:**

multiple sclerosis                obesity
cataracts                         swelling around the eyes
conjunctivitis                    fever
failure to thrive (in infants)    bed-wetting
diabetes                          low blood sugar
sneezing spells                   tinnitus
hoarseness                          (ringing of the ear)
otitis media (inflammation,
    discharge from ear, earaches)

The above list is not all-inclusive. More conditions are constantly being studied as possible allergic reactions to food and environmental chemicals. It is increasingly apparent that when allergy affects the central nervous system (brain and spinal cord), the result can be mood swings ranging from depression to manic-depressive and psychotic disorders and all the symptoms in between.

Already in 1931, Dr. Albert Rowe had published his book on the specific subject of food allergy. Dr. Rowe showed how food allergy was responsible for a wide range of symptoms which can affect any part of the body and can begin at any age. He also demonstrated that most people are affected by food allergy in varying degrees throughout their lives. Keeping in mind the hallmark signs of allergy – tissue redness, swelling, heat and pain – let's explore specific areas of the body that are commonly affected.

## The Gastrointestinal Tract

More symptoms of food allergy arise in the tissue of the gastrointestinal tract than in any other tissue of the body. Foods have direct contact for the longest time with the lining of the digestive tract, which can establish sensitization. This is especially true for the stomach, the duodenum (small intestine) and the rectum. Antibodies coat the mucosa (lining) of the gastrointestinal tract to act as a barrier to the external world.

When an allergic reaction occurs here, the released products such as histamine cause inflammation in the mucosa which becomes more permeable. Large particles (macromolecules) of incompletely digested food can then be absorbed through the mucosa and gain entrance to the blood stream. Once in the blood stream, these particles can be carried to any part of the body. Studies have shown that when the stomach has an absent or diminished supply of hydrochloric acid, even more macromolecules are found to be absorbed by the intestine, due to the fact that there are more particles present. Also, when trypsin, a pancreatic protein-digesting enzyme, is inhibited, more macromolecules are absorbed. Another study showed that low stomach acid results in increased formation of antibodies to cow's milk. The body reacts to macromolecules in the blood stream by producing more antibodies. Other ways the intestinal lining can become damaged are prolonged bacterial, viral, or yeast infection, parasites, toxins, decreased oxygen supply to the mucosa and X-radiation used in treating cancer.

Considering that one third of all surgery is for digestive diseases, it would seem prudent to explore the extent to which allergic reactions to food are involved. Digestive diseases are the second highest cause of doctor visits. Common intestinal conditions associated with food allergy are ulcers, sores in the mouth, colic, diarrhea, constipation, hemorrhoids, colitis and Crohn's disease.

**The Stomach:** Allergic reactions that occur in the stomach lead to the release of histamine from the mast cells lining the stomach. The histamine then triggers a large acid outpouring which can result in ulcer formation.

**Small Intestine and Colon:** Allergy to milk is by far the most frequent cause of chronic duodenal ulcers and colitis. Whenever these conditions exist dairy products should be suspected. Allergy to grain, especially wheat, is another common precipitator of intestinal distress.

## The Gall Bladder

Eating foods to which one is allergic can create gall bladder distress. The allergic reaction here causes swelling of the bile duct, which impairs emptying of the bile from the gall bladder into the small intestine. The accumulating fluid attracts infection and precipitates cholesterol, forming stones. Eggs have been shown to be the most common allergen affecting the gall bladder. Pork is also frequently involved, precipitating such severe symptoms that surgical removal of the gall bladder may result. In one study involving sixty-nine patients with gallstones, 92 percent reacted to egg, 63 percent reacted to pork, 52 percent reacted to onion, 34 percent reacted to fowl and 21 percent reacted to coffee.

## The Pancreas

When food is eaten, one of the first organs to be affected is the pancreas. If an allergic reaction to that food takes place, the pancreas can become the primary "shock organ." A "shock organ" is the site or tissue where an allergic reaction takes place.

The pancreas reacts first with over-stimulation. When over-stimulation is sustained long enough, inhibition or decreased function results. Production of bicarbonate, the alkaline fluid that neutralizes the stomach acid in the small intestine, is the first function to suffer. When the stomach acid is not neutralized, acid can be absorbed through the intestine and create an over-acid condition in the body. A common symptom of acidity is headaches.

The next function of the pancreas to be inhibited is the digestive enzyme production. These are the enzymes necessary to break down foods into absorbable products. A little-known function of proteolytic enzymes is that they also act as regulators of inflammatory reactions in the body. In other words, they can be used by the body to reduce or prevent inflammation. When proteolytic enzyme production is decreased, inflammatory kinins and prostaglandins can accumulate in ever-increasing quantity in the tissues, thus evoking inflammatory reactions throughout the body.

When not enough digestive enzymes are produced by the pancreas two major things happen. First, undigested fragments of food can be absorbed through the intestinal lining and into the blood stream. Antibodies recognize these particles as foreign invaders and attack, creating allergic reactions within the body. The less enzymes, the more undigested food particles there are in the intestine. The higher the concentration of these particles in the intestine, the more particles that can be absorbed into the blood.

Second, diminished enzyme output causes a lack of protein digestion: amino acids are the end products of protein digestion and when there are not enough proteolytic enzymes, the amino acid production suffers. *Antibodies, hormones and enzymes are all built from amino acids.* Insulin, needed for glucose metabolism, is made *entirely* from amino acids. The immune system is adversely affected due to lowered antibody production. Without sufficient amino acids, more digestive enzymes cannot be made, and a self-perpetuating, vicious cycle begins.

The last function of the pancreas to be affected by allergic reaction is insulin production. A lack of insulin is associated with diabetes.

## The Blood Vessels

Food reactions often create vast changes in arteries. These changes include spasms, swelling and dilation. In the temporal arteries, food reactions often cause constriction and edema, resulting in migraine. Vascular spasms have been implicated in some cases of epilepsy. If the coronary arteries are involved allergically, damage to the lining may occur, leading to cholesterol accumulation and myocardial infarction (heart attack).

## The Heart

The following symptoms have been seen in allergy affecting the heart: extra heartbeats, tachycardia (fast heartbeat), flutters, fibrillation, angina (pain), inflammation of the pericardium (sac surrounding the heart) and murmurs. These symptoms may result from allergic reactions to foods, tobacco, antibiotics or other drugs. Twenty-five percent of arrhythmias are triggered by food allergies.

## Hypoglycemia (blood sugar levels)

Unstable blood sugar, or hypoglycemia, can cause a wide range of symptoms similar to allergy such as fatigue, overweight, light headedness, confusion, frequent hunger pains, anxiety, nervousness, weakness, panic attacks and depression. In his book *Victory Over Diabetes,* Dr. William H. Philpott states that both high and low blood sugar can be seen in a person who has eaten any food or come in contact with any chemical to which he reacts allergically. In other words, any substance that can elicit an allergic reaction in an individual will raise or lower blood sugar levels, evoking symptoms of hypoglycemia.

The problem is not the type of food, such as sugar, that has traditionally been restricted in the diet of the hypoglycemic, but with the allergic reaction to a specific chemical or food. Dr. Philpott cites the following case of a man with diabetes: "I have observed for quite some time many diabetics who reacted very seriously to petrochemical hydrocarbons, such as found in exhaust fumes from cars, in perfumes or in fumes from natural gas. In Carl's case, a 30-minute test exposure to auto exhaust, as is usually experienced in city traffic, produced a shift in blood sugar from forty milligrams percent before exposure to well over a hundred and eighty milligrams percent after exposure." This example demonstrates that blood sugar levels can change dramatically due to contact with substances other than food!

## Obesity

Obesity usually involves addiction to several foods. Along with addictions come cravings and accompanying withdrawal effects. The foods you crave and eat the most often, or more than three times a week, are very likely to be your specific allergic foods. It is not a coincidence that the most frequently eaten foods are the most common allergens. Craving and insatiable hunger are characteristic symptoms of withdrawal. When the food is subsequently eaten, the person feels better – another tip-off of an addiction. Addiction is also indicated by the fact that when foods are spaced out or rotated on the basis of once every four to five days, there is a startling reduction in the hunger urge. If you have a craving for something sweet, especially following a meal, your blood sugar has probably dropped due to an allergic reaction to something you just ate. The mere elimination of foods to which a person reacts allergically results in about ten pounds of weight loss with no other dietary change.

Another interesting fact concerns lipase, the enzyme that digests fat. The lipase levels of fat cells in an obese person are much lower than the lipase levels of fat cells of a normal-weight individual. Lipase is necessary in the cell for the cell's fat to be mobilized and subsequently burned for energy. This indicates that an obese person may have a lipase deficiency, or exhausted lipase production.

## Musculoskeletal System

One of the more poorly recognized areas of allergy is its relation to the muscles and joints. Of all the muscle aches and pains, those in the muscles of the upper back, neck and shoulders are especially linked to diet and maladaptive or allergic reactions. Dr. Rowe observed muscle aches and pains to be part of a syndrome that he called "allergic toxemia." The main symptoms he observed were fatigue and headaches, drowsiness, mental confusion, slowness of thought, irritability, depression and *body aching*. Rowe was able to correlate specific foods to these symptoms. The patient may describe these symptoms as pulling and drawing sensations and stiffness or aching at the base of the neck. In the lower half of the body, the muscles most commonly affected are the hamstrings in the legs as well as the lower back muscles. Experiments have shown that these symptoms can all be reproduced by challenges with test foods or chemicals in susceptible persons. Instances of acute low back pain, acute bursitis and acute torticollis (stiff neck) are not uncommon. These aches, pains and stiffness are most common when a person first arises in the morning. If a person has recurring episodes and is otherwise chronically ill, allergies should be investigated.

## Arthritis (joints)

It is well established that joint symptoms do occur in people who have allergic symptoms. Dr. James C. Breneman found relief of arthritic symptoms in at least half of arthritic patients when their food allergens were identified and eliminated. Milk, wheat, egg, corn and pork were the most common food allergens. Doctors have long been aware of a relationship between gastrointestinal disease and arthritis. For example, a frequent side effect of intestinal bypass surgery is the development of a rheumatoid-type arthritis. Many gastrointestinal infections result in arthritis. Numerous studies show that arthritis can be produced at will in humans by feeding them foods to which they are allergic, and that the symptoms respond favorably when these foods are eliminated from the diet. It has been discovered that diet can precipitate arthritis in two ways: by either being deficient in nutrients, or by containing nutrients the body is not able to absorb and use. This paves the way for the second stage, allergic reactions.

The status of food allergy as a precipitative agent in rheumatoid arthritis has been demonstrated on numerous occasions since 1949. More recently, arthritis and environmental chemical pollutants have been investigated and have been found to have a high correlation. Theron G. Randolph, MD found that "With but rare exceptions, cases of rheumatoid arthritis now respond favorably to the avoidance of incriminated foods and chemical exposures including air pollutants, food and water additives and contaminants and synthetically derived or chemically contaminated drugs." He reports that when patients were fasted and then challenged with specific foods that symptoms developed. A typical case from his report is given below, in which the patient was fasted and then challenged with the following foods:

| | | |
|---|---|---|
| corn | 10 mins. | Severe arthritic pain |
| cane sugar | 15 mins. | Pains in knees and hands plus abdominal cramps |
| apple | 30 mins. | Abdominal distress and arthritis |
| lamb | 35 mins. | Severe arthritis |
| orange | 40 mins. | Intermittent waves of apprehension and depression followed by progressively severe arthritis |

The January 1980 issue of *Annals of Allergy* reported a study involving subjects with both osteoarthritis and rheumatoid arthritis, the two main types of arthritic disease. Eighty-seven percent of the test subjects were found to have allergies that could cause such common symptoms as swelling and pain. Dr. James C. Breneman considers joint pain to be a very late manifestation of a food allergy reaction. He further states that, "The immunological etiology of arthritis seems well established." Part of the problem, he reports, is that often the joint pains may not appear for 42 to 72 hours after exposure to the allergic food. In the case of reaction to pork, symptoms may not appear for five days.

## Upper Respiratory Infections

The nasal and sinus membranes are very sensitive to allergic irritants. These irritants do not have to be inhaled. They can also be foods to which a person is allergic. Once the membranes are irritated and swollen they are easily infected by bacteria or viruses, or they can become reactive to pollens and dust. These edematous tissues become chronically infected by repeated exposure to foods or inhalants that trigger allergic reactions.

## Asthma (lungs)

Mast cells line the bronchi (the tubes leading from the trachea to the lungs). When the cells encounter an allergen, they release inflammatory products which cause inflammation in the tissues. This irritation produces muscular contractions, which restrict air flow through the bronchial passage. Common irritants include tobacco smoke, chemical fumes, very cold air, bacterial infections, aspirin, sulfites and MSG (monosodium glutamate), but any food or air pollutant can be involved. The most common foods involved in asthma are milk, egg, wheat, seafood, peanuts and nuts.

## Nephrosis (kidney disease)

Studies show that children with nephrosis are made significantly worse when fed their individual food allergens. Proteinuria (protein in the urine) improved when the allergens were eliminated from the diet.

## Adrenal Glands

People exhibiting multiple allergies – thirty or more – often have weakened adrenal glands. The adrenal glands are important because they produce hormones such as cortisone which helps to prevent or decrease the intensity of allergic reactions. Excessive ingestion of white sugar and white flour products and other refined foods stress the adrenal glands. People with weakened adrenals tend to crave salt.

## Headache

In cases where headaches are caused by allergenic foods, symptoms usually appear within an hour of consumption. Fatigue is considered the most frequent allergic symptom, however headache runs a close second. It makes more sense to investigate headache from the standpoint of its possible environmental cause than to treat it with painkillers. The most common foods reported to be involved in headache are milk, chocolate, peanuts, pork, egg and coffee. According to many researchers, food allergy is the number one cause of migraine headache. Leon Unger, MD and Joel Cristol, MD reported in their article "Allergic Migraines" which appeared in the *Annals of Allergy* that migraine headache is an allergic disease caused by one or more foods. Many prominent researchers have since supported this view.

## Fatigue

Fatigue is the number one allergic sign. It tends to be worse in the morning and again in late afternoon. No amount of rest relieves the tiredness.

## Diagnosing Allergy

Because of the widely varying manifestations of allergy in the many tissues of the body, developing valid tests for allergy has been a challenge. Nevertheless, many different diagnostic tests have been devised. All of them have their own strengths and weaknesses. A good patient history is still considered to be the best indicator of an allergic condition. As with most diagnostic tests, the value of tests for allergy depends on the knowledge of their interpreter. Some of the more common tests used to detect allergy are described below.

**Skin Testing:** The basic method is pricking the skin to deliver a solution of allergen under the skin. The skin is then observed for various degrees of swelling and redness.

While this is one of the most widely used tests to identify allergy, it works best for only certain types of allergy, especially inhalant allergy. Where food allergy is concerned, it may not produce a positive result simply because the required IgE antibody is not found in the skin. In this case, the IgE may be localized to some other tissue such as the intestine or nose, and it has not entered the general circulation (blood stream), which is the reason it is not present in the skin.

**RAST (Radioallergosorbent Test):** The RAST is a blood test which requires the presence of an IgE antibody to detect allergy. This test is more expensive to administer than skin testing.

**Cytotoxic Test:** In this test white blood cells are mixed with a food extract. When subsequent changes to the white blood cells are observed, the test is positive for that food.

**Elimination-Provocation:** This test is the most widely accepted by the medical community. The patient is either fasted on water only or given a hypoallergenic diet for five days to one week. Then foods are reintroduced one at a time and the patient is observed for reactions (symptoms). The main disadvantage to this test is, of course, the time involved. It can take days or weeks.

**Sublingual Provocation:** This test is performed by placing a test substance under the tongue. Then a major muscle is tested for a change in muscle strength. Weakening of the muscle when challenged with the test substance is an indication of sensitivity to that substance.

Dr. George Goodheart, the developer of applied kinesiology, pioneered the study of the connection between a substance placed under the patient's tongue and alterations in muscle strength. When an allergen or substance that an individual is sensitive to is placed in the mouth, there is an immediate and measurable weakening of that individual's muscle strength.

Dr. Hugh Cox, a founder of the British Society of Clinical Ecology, extended this work by taking a dilution of a food concentrate rather than the actual food, placing it under the patient's tongue and observing changes in muscle strength. In subsequent tests, he injected the dilution of the food concentrate under the skin to produce a skin reaction, such as a welt or flare on the skin surface. This is similar to the familiar skin prick test for allergy. Dr. Cox noticed that when the same dilution that caused a skin reaction was placed under the patient's tongue, it would produce dramatically weakened muscle responses. This is an objective and precise correlation between the two methods of testing. Dr. Cox further experimented by placing the drops on the skin itself. He got an identical weak muscle response. These weakened responses were later confirmed in double blind studies. Dr. Cox believes that when the body comes in contact with an allergen, the electrical potential of the allergen interferes with the electrical firing of the motor endplate of the muscle, thereby producing the muscle changes.

# 7

# Addiction and Allergy

*A*ddiction plays a role in allergy. As a general rule, what you crave is what you are allergic to. This is illustrated in the following example.

Louise arrives home after an especially long day at work. Feeling tired and stressed, she greets her children briefly before heading for the kitchen to start dinner. As she is taking a casserole from the refrigerator to the oven, she spies some dinner rolls she made the previous day. Louise quickly heats one in the microwave and devours it. She feels instantly better. Is this an addiction? If instead Louise had reached for a cocktail or a glass of wine, would that be an addiction? The answer is that either could be an addiction, depending on certain factors.

We tend to think of addiction in terms of substances such as drugs, caffeine, tobacco and alcohol. But is it possible to be addicted to foods such as wheat, cheese or pickles? What are the signs? Addiction goes hand in hand with allergy. With foods, addiction can be either conscious or subconscious. Your favorite foods are usually the ones that you are allergic to and are also addicted to.

Do you crave a certain food frequently? Do you eat it even though you don't feel so good the next day? Do you feel immediately better upon eating a certain food? If the answer is yes, you may be addicted. Addiction causes chronic symptoms often hours or days after the food is eaten. Some of these symptoms include fatigue, weakness, headaches, irritability and depression. When the addictive food is eaten again, the symptoms disappear temporarily. However, a person can often keep himself in a symptom-free state by eating the addictive food frequently, thereby postponing symptoms of withdrawal. The result is that there is chronic stress to the body, eventually leading to chronic and degenerative disease.

The book *Clinical Ecology* reports that, "Food addiction has the same characteristics of relief on exposure and emergence of delayed reactions as has addiction to tobacco, narcotics or alcohol." It is possible to be addicted to anything, including common foods and chemicals such as in perfume and hair spray. Foods are the primary potential addictants for three reasons:

1. The sheer bulk of food: large amounts are eaten – two to five pounds per day.
2. Frequency: food is eaten daily, several times a day.
3. Intimacy or duration of exposure: food stays in contact with the digestive tract for a long time.

Withdrawal reactions last four to five days when an addictive food is removed from the diet. Eating the food after withholding it from the diet for four to five days will cause an increased allergic reaction. This is the basis for using the elimination diet as a diagnostic test.

The increased reaction is probably due to the fact that the immune system has had four to five days to strengthen or recuperate while the food was removed.

There are four cardinal signs of addiction:

1. Obsession: the person often cannot stop thinking about food. He plans the next time he will eat it. When he is close to getting the food, he may feel an anxiety or excitement that does not let up until he actually eats the food. He arranges his life in ways that will facilitate him obtaining the food.
2. Negative consequences: the person will eat the food, in spite of the fact that it may have negative consequences. For instance, a person eats six candy bars even though he knows he will feel bloated, tired and unable to do more than watch television that evening. Addictive behaviors produce pleasure, relief and other payoffs that ignore harmful consequences.

3. Lack of control: do you know anyone who, once he eats the first doughnut, cannot stop until the whole box is gone? Or he eats a potato chip and cannot stop until the whole bag is empty? Inability to control or stop the behavior is a mark of addiction. When the person tries to bring the behavior under control, willpower alone is not enough. The food is controlling him rather than the other way around.

4. Denial: denying that a food can be the cause of your burning stomach, aching shoulders or swollen joints is characteristic of addiction. You dismiss obvious symptoms by saying: "I didn't eat very much of it," or, "My doctor says it can't possibly be the cause of my colitis," or avoiding the subject altogether.

Why, you might wonder, are the most commonly eaten foods such as milk, wheat, egg and corn also the foods most frequently found to be allergenic? The answer lies in understanding enzyme deficiency. When you eat a food frequently, such as milk on your breakfast cereal, a glass of milk for lunch, an ice cream cone in the afternoon and milk in the form of cheese on your pizza for dinner, you are calling on specific enzymes to digest that milk. When this eating pattern continues over days, weeks and years, you may create an enzyme deficiency for that food. The same is true for wheat. When you eat wheat in the form of toast or pancakes or doughnuts for breakfast, wheat in the bread of your sandwich for lunch and wheat in dinner rolls or in breaded fried chicken in the evening, specific enzymes are called on over and over until they are eventually depleted. Milk and wheat are the two most common allergenic foods and they are often eaten together: cereal and milk, cheese sandwich, cheeseburger with a glass of milk and pizza with a wheat crust and cheese are common examples. This stresses the enzyme systems even more.

Anything consumed on a daily basis is a potential allergen. Corn is another good example. A person may not eat corn itself, but he may still be consuming great quantities of corn daily in the form of corn oil, corn starch, corn syrup, cereal, dextrin, corn meal or alcohol made from corn. By 1967, one hundred and thirty supermarket products contained some form of corn. All chemical and ingested food allergies and addictions eventually lead to pancreatic injury.

With a compromised pancreas production of bicarbonate – needed to neutralize stomach acid – and production of enzymes are the most affected. Through allergy and addiction, foods can harm your health over a period of time.

*Clinical Ecology* states, "Allergic and allergic-like maladaptive reactions have been so characterized by the fact that immediate and/or relatively immediate reactions occur on exposure. Addiction has been characterized by an initial relief, or partial relief, on exposure and the emergence of delayed reactions which can again be relieved by exposure." Common withdrawal symptoms from food are:

1. Feeling of having influenza.
2. Aching of all parts of the body.
3. High temperature or fever.
4. Severe headaches.
5. Palpitations.
6. Pains in parts of the body that have not been affected before.

Withdrawal effects have been known to persist for as long as 20 hours when an allergic food is eaten only once per 24 hours. When the allergic food is eaten three times a day, symptoms are most likely to be noticed first thing upon arising in the morning.

It is easier to become addicted to a refined, processed food than to a whole food in its natural state. A refined food has lost its normal protective ratios of synergistic vitamins, minerals and enzymes either by removal or destruction. This alters the way the refined food is metabolized in the body. For example, sugar acts more like a drug in the body than like a food because it has been refined to a "pure" form, devoid of its complementary nutrients. In its natural state, as sugar cane, it supplies B vitamins and many trace minerals including chromium. When refined sugar is eaten, these nutrients must be supplied from body stores in order for the sugar to be metabolized. If these nutrient stores are depleted, alternate metabolic pathways of the body must be used, which can create an imbalance in the body's biochemistry. This imbalance results in altered signals to the brain, leading to craving and addiction. Eating whole foods in the natural state has been shown clinically to be the quickest way to eliminate cravings.

# 8

# Yeasts, Molds and Parasites

With increased understanding of how allergy arises, how it affects the tissues, how it is recognized and what symptoms it can produce, let's explore other factors that dramatically affect allergy.

Infections by yeasts, molds and parasites have an important connection to allergy and are frequently found in individuals suffering from allergy. The most common organism in this category is *Candida albicans*.

## Candida albicans

*Candida albicans,* a yeast, sets the stage for allergy. When this yeast is present as a systemic infection in a person, it is virtually impossible for that person to get well from allergy unless he first brings the Candida infection under control. This is because *Candida albicans* keeps the immune system in an impoverished state and a healthy immune system is required to eliminate allergies.

It is estimated that sixty million Americans have systemic yeast infection. *Candida albicans* is normally present in the colon along with at least four hundred other types of organisms. Only when it grows out of balance in relationship to those other organisms is it able to proliferate in the body and spread to other tissues. At least 80 species of the Candida organism have been identified and so far at least six of them have been implicated as human pathogens.

When Candida proliferates in the body, the condition is referred to as an overgrowth syndrome. This syndrome, also called candidiasis, is created in the body in a number of different ways. The most common cause is the overuse of antibiotics. Antibiotics used frequently or over a long period of time, such as tetracycline for acne, help create candidiasis. Antibiotics kill off the necessary, "friendly" bacteria that serve to keep the yeast in check. These friendly bacteria keep Candida in balance by competing for food and by producing the B vitamin, biotin, which helps to block yeast overgrowth. Use of steroids such as cortisone also invites various infections.

Birth control pills create hormonal imbalances that serve to encourage yeast growth and *Candida albicans* itself can interfere with hormonal function in the body. Birth control pills contain steroid hormones. Candida has a steroid-binding protein, which means that the yeast is able to take the steroid into its own cellular structure. The Candida can then participate in and interfere with human hormonal signal systems. Candida binds even more efficiently with corticosteroids and progesterone.

Laboratory studies done on rats indicate that the Candida glycoproteins can stimulate histamine release from the mast cells. These are the cells involved in classic allergic reactions. Histamine creates membrane permeability, and when histamine is released on a continual basis it can be carried throughout the body, affecting tissues anywhere. Babies can be born with Candida infection since the organism can cross the placental barrier *in utero*.

Diets high in processed foods and sugar favor Candida growth. Even the chlorine added to tap water plays a role as it tends to upset the normal bacterial flora of the intestine. As you can see, anything that upsets the normal flora of the intestine will encourage Candida growth.

Candida can exist in two forms. The form that is normally seen in the colon is in the sugar-fermenting or actively reproducing state. In this form it is non-invasive. It does not migrate to other tissues. However, when it changes into its fungal form, it is able to penetrate the cells of the intestine and infiltrate other tissues of the body. In this invasive form, Candida is thought to grow mycelia, which are thread-like structures that can penetrate cells and extract nutrients. This can cause the intestine to become more permeable, which then leads to allergies.

Once Candida migrates to other tissues, it can grow unchecked and produce toxins that have systemic effects. These toxins are capable of suppressing and inhibiting the immune system. One such toxin is acetaldehyde, a relative of formaldehyde. Acetaldehyde can cause several metabolic problems. It interferes with acetylcholine, a chemical found at nerve endings, changing normal transmission of impulses or information.

Yeast cells also appear to be able to produce hormone-like substances which stimulate estrogen production in the body. In this way yeast cells can interfere with normal hormonal communication, causing inappropriate signals to be sent. As a consequence, the immune system suffers. Some reports indicate that Candida also produces alcohol in the system. People in whom this occurs may appear to be drunk or mentally confused without ever taking a drink.

A little known fact is that Candida is a polyantigenic organism. This means there have been 79 immunological allergic characteristics isolated for *Candida albicans* at the present time. This can keep the immune system busy forming antibodies to the point of immune suppression or breakdown.

CASE STUDY: *Joan*

Joan, age 25, was bothered by hair falling out, creating a patch of missing hair on one side of her head. She also had pain in her right hip and lower abdomen. She was taking birth control pills, B vitamins and calcium.

Examination revealed that Joan had blood sugar instability and systemic Candida overgrowth. She was allergic to wheat, milk, fish, shellfish, nuts and cheese. Although she was supplementing with calcium, she was deficient in both calcium and magnesium. She also had a copper toxicity.

Joan was experiencing an inflammatory kinin reaction in her right lower abdomen whenever she ate meat. This reaction was also causing pain in her right hip. Enzyme therapy resolved this situation within two weeks. She was put on a program to clear the Candida overgrowth infection and reduce the copper toxicity. She was also given trace minerals and vitamins A, C and E. She received chiropractic adjustments to help strengthen and balance her structure and weak organs.

Most of Joan's symptoms cleared up within the first three weeks. However, her program was continued for three months to give all the tissues time to heal and strengthen, and to prevent recurrence. After that time, Joan did not require nutrient supplements. She also discontinued her birth control pills as she felt that they had contributed to her Candida infection.

Candidiasis is recognized as a polysymptomatic disease. This means that a person will exhibit a whole list of symptoms, many of which may seem bizarre. The person is often labeled as neurotic, or hypochondriac. Sometimes the yeast overgrowth is so severe that the person is hospitalized for mental illness. Some of the most common symptoms of candidiasis include fatigue, headaches, loss of energy, changing moods, bloating, abdominal gas and pain, heartburn, constipation, diarrhea, pain and swelling in the joints, nasal congestion, sinus problems, recurrent sore throat, ear itching, fluid in the ears, general malaise, vaginal itching and burning, tightness in the chest and forgetfulness. Symptoms tend to worsen on damp, rainy days and in places where molds can be inhaled. Symptoms can increase when candidiasis is combined with breathing in of chemicals such as tobacco smoke, perfumes, car exhaust and other pollutants.

Nearly one hundred Candida toxins have so far been identified. Two of them, carbon monoxide and acetylaldehyde, are known to be able to suppress the T-cells of the immune system – the fighter or "killer cells." Candida toxins create vascular permeability and enhance histamine release, both of which play roles in allergic reactions. As mentioned earlier, it is thought that acetylaldehyde produces central nervous system symptoms through its interference with nerve transmissions. Red blood cell flexibility is also lost when acetylaldehyde is present. This decreases the rate at which red blood cells can carry oxygen to the tissues. Since the brain is very oxygen-dependent, central nervous system symptoms may be created by this mechanism. Mood swings, irritability, behavioral changes and headaches are common symptoms of central nervous system involvement.

## CASE STUDY: *Tony*

Tony, age seven, weighed only 38 pounds and had not gained weight for several months. When I first saw him in my office, he displayed eczema which had been on his arms and legs since birth. He had frequent nosebleeds, gas, frequent infections and listlessness. He was also still wetting his bed at night.

Upon testing Tony was found to be reactive to milk, sugar, yeast and grain dust. His pituitary, thymus and pancreas were stressed and underactive. His mother had taken him for numerous medical examinations with no results. The only medication he was receiving at the time was a cortisone ointment that his mother said was not helping.

This patient was born with systemic Candida infection, which led to the multiplicity of his problems. He was put on a program to correct this condition and given *Lactobacillus acidophilus* to reculture the colon. He received chiropractic adjustments, concentrated plant enzymes and nutrient supplements to strengthen his immune system. The allergenic foods were eliminated from his diet.

Within two weeks, there was marked improvement in the eczema. Where the sores had been oozing red and raised above the skin level, they were now less red, flush with the skin, and did not itch. One month later, Tony was free of the eczema except for a small spot inside each elbow. The nosebleeds and bed-wetting had ceased.

However, at about this time, Tony developed a fever and swollen testicles. He was given antibiotics under medical therapy. The rash returned on his legs. When the course of antibiotics ran out, nutritional therapy was continued and the rash again disappeared. One year later all symptoms were gone and Tony had gained 15 pounds. He was now eating all foods except milk.

The symptoms of candidiasis often masquerade as symptoms of either allergy or hypoglycemia. These nearly identical symptoms link together the three conditions: candidiasis, hypoglycemia and allergy.

A person may have only one of these conditions at a time, or they may be seen together in a combined form. Those persons most severely ill with allergy have all three. It is estimated that 30 percent of the world's population has systemic candidiasis. Among patients with multiple allergies, however, the percentage goes up sharply. It has been found clinically that 80 percent of people with multiple allergies will have Candida overgrowth.

Increased antibiotic use in recent years appears to have contributed to the epidemic increase in candidiasis in North America. There are thousands of different antibiotics in use today. In fact, a dictionary of antibiotics alone has been published. Of course, it is not the antibiotics themselves that are the problem, but their widespread use and overuse that have created this sorry plight.

Many people are sure that they have not had antibiotics in any great amount. However, antibiotics are often present in today's meat supply. Almost all poultry, 70 percent of cattle and 90 percent of pigs raised commercially in the United States are ingesting antibiotics with their feed. Some residues of these antibiotics appear to remain in the meat and are transferable to humans when the meat is eaten.

Candida also has the ability to convert the mercury vapor from mercury in silver amalgam dental fillings to methyl mercury. Studies show mercury can be retained in brain tissue for 18 to 22 years.

A common sign of Candida infection is intolerance of cheese, wine and beer. If you get obvious symptoms after ingesting these products, you probably have systemic candidiasis and/or allergy to Candida or other yeasts.

In summary, the points to remember are:

1. Allergic patients frequently have Candida infection.
2. Candida produces toxins that impair the immune system.
3. The Candida organism itself can be an allergen.
4. Candida can damage the intestine and promote allergies.

## Molds

Molds which are inhaled, eaten or otherwise contacted pack a double punch. Not only are they capable of producing substances that are toxic to the nerves and particularly to the central nervous system, but an individual may also be allergic to the specific mold. When both these conditions are present, the symptoms are magnified.

A characteristic of molds is that they produce antibiotics, which they release into the surrounding environment to kill competing bacteria in the vicinity. These fungal products are capable of damaging tissue cells, especially nerves.

For example, the antibiotic cycloserine can cause hyper-irritability, aggression, psychosis, drowsiness, loss of memory, seizures, paralysis, convulsions and/or coma. These symptoms are clinically indistinguishable from the symptoms caused by psychic trauma.

Clinically, challenge tests with molds have produced the following symptoms: depression, weakness, fatigue, anger, confusion, fear, dizziness, anxiety, irritability, hostility, headaches, hyperactivity and inability to concentrate. Some forms of the mold aspergillis can reside in the chest for years contributing to breathing problems and asthma. These symptoms are recounted to increase awareness that mold allergy and mold toxins are capable of eliciting mild to severe mental and physical changes in a person.

Molds are known to produce symptoms three ways:

1. Molds give off toxins.
2. The immune system can produce antibodies which lead to allergic reactions to a specific mold.
3. Molds cause an increase in the number and intensity of allergic reactions to foods and chemicals.

## Parasites

Probably no other factor has been so overlooked by doctors in North America as the incidence of parasites. This is in spite of the fact that the World Health Organization estimates that there are 1.2 billion people with roundworm, 1 billion with hookworm and 700 million with tapeworm worldwide. Although many of these statistics reflect high levels of infestation in underdeveloped countries, it is becoming evident that parasitic infestation is far more common in North America than previously suspected. Regardless of the type of parasite that resides in the tissues, the end result of this parasitic infection is toxicity, tissue damage and immune system suppression.

Giardia is a parasite that is found throughout the world, especially in the tropics. However, it has become increasingly common in North America. Giardia produces hard-walled cysts that can get into food or water. These cysts are resistant to chlorine in the amount generally found in water supplies.

Diarrhea, bloating, abdominal pain, belching and fatigue are common symptoms upon initial infection. These symptoms subside after a few days. However, the infected person may remain infectious, capable of passing the infection to others. In the chronic state of Giardia infection, gas, abdominal bloating, belching, nausea, hives, joint pain and fever are common symptoms.

All chronic parasitic infections tend to lead to allergic states in the body since they overwork the immune system. Many also give off poisonous waste products which alter body functions. When lodged in a specific tissue, parasites can damage or destroy that tissue. The first step for anyone with allergies is to be checked thoroughly for yeast, molds and parasites.

# 9

# Acid-Base Balance is Critical

*A*llergy involves inflammation of the tissues, which causes tissue injury. These damaged tissues must heal. But what conditions does the body require in order to heal or repair these injured tissues? One of the most important but least understood conditions affecting the healing process is the acid-base balance of the body. Not only is the proper pH of the body essential to healing, it is essential to prevent further allergic reactions.

Guyton's *Textbook of Medical Physiology* states that regulation of the pH of the body is one of the most important aspects of homeostasis. What is pH? It is a measure of the acidity or alkalinity of a substance on a scale which runs from 0 to 14 with 7 being neutral. Neutral is neither acid nor alkaline. Zero is totally acid and 14 totally alkaline. In between are varying degrees of acidity and alkalinity.

The blood in the human body is at a pH of 7.4, which is slightly alkaline. If the pH of the blood were to make as small a change as to 6.8, which is barely acid, severe consequences such as coma would result. The heart would relax and then stop beating. If the pH of the blood were to increase to just 8.0, tetanic convulsions would occur and the heart would cease to beat. According to Guyton's *Textbook of Medical Physiology*, "Only slight changes in hydrogen ion concentration from the normal value can cause marked alteration in the rate of chemical reactions in the cells, some being depressed and others

65

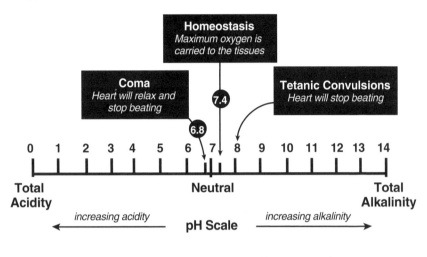

The blood must remain within a narrow pH range around 7.4.
The body gives blood pH priority over other body functions:
The heart will stop beating if the blood pH lowers to 6.8 or rises to 8.0.

*Figure 2.* **Blood pH Range**

accelerated." Since life-threatening conditions can occur with only small changes in the blood pH, the body will do whatever is necessary to maintain a constant blood pH of 7.4. Survival depends on the blood remaining at the slightly alkaline pH of 7.4.

When the blood shows a slight degree of acidity, a greater swing toward acidity at the cellular level usually occurs. As the blood is pushed by stimuli in an acid direction, it will buffer this acid with alkalizing minerals from other tissues. These minerals include potassium, sodium, calcium and magnesium. Once used, these minerals can be replaced in the body only by foods – particularly the alkaline fruits and vegetables.

Fruits and vegetables contribute minerals to your body in the following manner. Organic acids, such as those found in citrus fruits and most vegetables, contain the alkalizing minerals sodium, potassium, calcium and magnesium. When oxidized, these organic acids become carbon dioxide and water, which are eliminated through the lungs and kidneys. The alkaline minerals remain behind and neutralize body acids (acid waste from cell metabolism). This is why most

66

fruits and vegetables are considered to be alkaline-forming foods. They are mineral donors.

The sodium that the body requires cannot come from the sodium found in table salt (sodium chloride). The reason is that table salt has tight ionic bonds which are difficult for the body to break apart. Table salt has been heated to over 500°F in the refining process, making those bonds even tighter. The body can easily use sodium with loose covalent bonds, such as is found in raw fruits and vegetables. These foods are the main suppliers of sodium to the body.

The typical recommendation to cut back on salt is good advice when it comes to processed foods and table salt. However, sodium from natural fruits and vegetables is an essential nutrient and plays a major role in the body.

Sodium drives the sodium-potassium pump in every cell of the body. The main function of this pump is to produce energy in the form of ATP (adenosine triphosphate). Without sufficient sodium, energy production decreases. Fatigue is the result. Sodium and potassium are necessary for this vital body function, as well as for neutralizing the acids of the body.

In allergic conditions, slight changes in acid-base metabolism occur. Excess acidity depletes the body's stores of minerals. Having less minerals lowers the body's ability to make enzymes since minerals are necessary for enzyme production and for carrying electrical currents in the body. Eating more alkalizing foods such as fruits and vegetables helps restore minerals to the body and promotes healing.

In addition, excess acidity causes the activity of the cells to slow down. When this happens, fatigue results. Fatigue is the number one symptom in most degenerative conditions including allergy.

## Are You Solar Powered?

In the numerous books written on "healing foods," "energy foods" and "high energy diets," raw fruits and vegetables play the starring role. Why is this? Why don't these books recommend "power" cereals and "big beef" meals?

Are fruits and vegetables different from these other forms of food? They are in the sense that only plant life can pick up and use energy from the sun through a process called photosynthesis. The carbon dioxide that we breath out as a waste product is "breath" for the plants which take in carbon dioxide, release oxygen and store solar energy in chemical form. When we eat these plants, the oxygen we have taken in releases the plants' stored energy to our cells. This is one reason why, when a person goes on a raw food diet, he nearly always notices a burst of energy. If you are suffering from fatigue, perhaps you need a little more "solar power."

Remember, when the cells are impaired, the ability of each cell to produce energy is diminished. How do our modern diets relate to acid-base balance? We find some rather shocking news. In the last 50 years fruit and vegetable consumption has decreased by 40 to 45 percent. At the same time fat, salt and sugar consumption has increased by 100 percent. Whole grain consumption has decreased substantially, while consumption of bakery goods has increased by 70 percent. These changes are due to the increased production and availability of refined, processed and fast foods.

Fruits and vegetables are the body's main source of minerals or alkaline elements. A diet lacking fruits and vegetables and containing excess meat, fat and refined products will constantly push the body pH toward the acid state. This type of diet does three things:

1. It supplies many acid-forming factors.
2. It fails to contribute alkaline-forming elements.
3. It uses up the body's stored minerals by requiring excessive quantities of them to neutralize acids.

Stimulating the body continuously in one direction has the effect of eventually exhausting the body systems. The body will then change its functions in order to adapt to the new situation. These adaptations in function eventually lead to degenerative changes in tissues, organs and bony structures.

Diet is the largest single stimulus to the body's biochemical balance or homeostasis. Whatever you put in the body, the body must deal with, and you can drive your body in either an acid or alkaline direction over a period of time. Dr. M. Ted Morter Jr. explains, "Disease is a by-product of lowered resistance. Lowered resistance is a by-product of an unfavorable internal environment. An unfavorable internal environment is brought about principally by putting the wrong things into the body for it to work with." Let's look at each of these "wrong things": excess protein, excess fat and refined foods.

## Excess Protein

The average American eats 80 to 125 grams of protein per day. This is twice the Recommended Daily Allowance (RDA) for protein intake. The RDA recommends 63 grams for mature males and 50 grams for mature females. The RDA recommendations for protein have decreased over the last 20 years and many doctors feel the RDA for protein could be even lower.

Guyton's *Textbook of Medical Physiology* tells us that 20 to 30 grams of protein replaces the protein used up by the body daily. It suggests that an average person can maintain normal protein stores with a daily intake of 30 to 55 grams. Protein is continuously being broken down and re-synthesized by the body. The *Recommended Dietary Allowances* (RDA), 10th edition, states, "Several times more protein is turned over daily within the body than is ordinarily consumed indicating that re-utilization of amino acids is a major factor of the economy of protein metabolism." The same volume tells us that protein deficiency, besides being rare, does not occur in an isolated condition, but rather as a consequence of total calorie deprivation. In other words, it is difficult to have a protein deficiency in the absence of total starvation.

Some people feel they need to increase protein intake to compensate for vigorous exercise. This is not true according to the RDA. "There is little evidence that muscular activity increases the need for protein except for the small amount required for the development of muscles during physical conditioning." The RDA further states that, "In the view of the margin of safety in the RDA no increment is added for work or training." The authors of the RDA have already added an extra amount of protein to what studies show is actually required, making it unnecessary to include more protein for work. This "margin of safety" means that extra protein for work has already been included even though you may be sedentary.

How much is 30 grams of protein?

| Food Source | Protein Content |
| --- | --- |
| 6 chicken nuggets | 20 g protein |
| Big Mac | 25 g protein |
| Quarter Pounder with Cheese | 28 g protein |
| two slices of pepperoni pizza | 26 g protein |
| a beef burrito | 25 g protein |
| taco salad with the shell | 34 g protein |
| 4 oz. American cheese | 24 g protein |
| 4 oz. cheddar cheese | 28 g protein |
| 1 cup whole milk | 8 g protein |
| 4 oz. almonds | 20 g protein |
| 1 egg | 6 g protein |
| 4 oz. broiled chicken | 33 g protein |
| 4 oz. broiled fresh flounder | 27 g protein |
| 4 oz. hamburger | 20 g protein |
| 1/2 cup boiled pinto beans | 7 g protein |
| 1/2 cup boiled kidney beans | 6 g protein |

The acids produced from excess protein must be neutralized to prevent them from harming the body. In accomplishing this, the alkaline minerals sodium, calcium and potassium are used. If excess protein must be continuously neutralized over a long period of time, the body's alkaline reserve is depleted. So what should be done? The message here is not to stop eating protein altogether. Protein is absolutely essential for health. It is the *excess* protein that creates problems and toxicity in the body, stressing alkaline reserves. You must know how much protein you are consuming and keep the amount to a healthful level.

As you can see, only a small amount of protein is actually required daily. How many people sit down to an eight ounce (64 g) or 12 ounce (96 g) steak for dinner and consume that in only one meal? Perhaps they also had bacon (6 g per 3 slices) and eggs (12 g per 2 eggs) for breakfast and a hamburger (24 g) for lunch. That would be a total of 138 g.

Excess protein can create dangerous conditions in the body. Most animal proteins supply sulfur and phosphorus. Phosphorus is abundant in animal-source foods and can produce poisonous acid. When animal protein is metabolized, sulphur and phosphorus form sulfuric and phosphoric acid which must be neutralized by the alkaline body minerals before they can be excreted by the kidneys. This is the reason animal foods are considered to be acid-forming foods.

Furthermore, excess protein breaks down to produce urea which has a diuretic effect causing both water and valuable minerals such as calcium, sodium and potassium to be lost in the urine. Since these minerals are alkaline-forming elements, the result of excess protein is to push the body toward the acid state.

Excess protein can also change the pH of the fluids surrounding the cells, thereby upsetting the osmotic balance of the cells. The osmotic balance is the pressure between the fluids on either side of the cell membrane. When the pH of these fluids changes water may flow into the cells. Protein synthesis inside the cell can be impaired by alterations of the pH of the fluid surrounding the cell.

All functions in the body are dependent upon the pH balance. However, of particular interest is how white blood cell production depends upon the acid-base balance. When the body is pushed toward the acid side, white blood cell production is lowered. This, of course, interferes with the immune system which relies on its white blood cells.

How does all this relate to allergy? *Clinical Ecology* tells us, "Maladaptive symptoms quickly develop when the pH is not optimum." Monitoring pH at the time that maladaptive symptoms develop reveals that acidification is characteristic. Many allergic reactions not only occur in, but help to create acid conditions in the body. *Clinical Ecology* goes on to say that it takes a very strong stimulus for a healthy person to develop symptoms. "A biologically healthy organism will develop symptoms on exposure to overwhelmingly strong stimuli. A biologically defective organism, due to an irritable or over-responsive central nervous system, will develop symptoms to normal or even subnormal stimuli."

Many symptoms develop when the body is in a slightly acid state. These symptoms include fatigue, pain, stomach pain, chest pain, frequent sighing, allergies, insomnia, water retention, arthritis, migraine headaches, low blood pressure, dry hard stools, alternating constipation and diarrhea, difficulty swallowing, burning in the mouth and/or under the tongue, bumps on the roof of the mouth or tongue and aches and pains on arising which improve as the day goes on.

Symptoms which occur when the body is in a slightly alkaline state include sore muscles, creaking joints, bursitis, bone spurs, drowsiness, hypertension, hypothermia (low body temperature), edema, allergies, night cramps, asthma, chronic indigestion, night coughs, vomiting, menstrual problems, hard dry stools, prostatitis and skin itching. In the absence of major pathology, the primary cause of alkalosis is the taking of antacids for digestive complaints.

One study showed that when grain was chewed one hundred to two hundred times per mouthful, the grain became alkaline by mixing with the alkaline salivary enzyme ptyalin and thus did not create acidity. The blood can most easily stay at the slightly alkaline pH of 7.4 when alkaline foods predominate in the diet. A blood pH of 7.4 creates a healing environment and regeneration at the cellular level. If you give the body what it needs, it can do the necessary repair. In general, fruits and vegetables are alkalizing and meats and grains are acidifying.

## Excess Fat

Fats have an acidifying effect because excess fat tends to block oxygen from reaching the cells. With less oxygen, the sodium-potassium pump of the cell slows down and waste products start to accumulate in the cell. These waste products are acidic. In addition, excess fat is often incompletely broken down by the digestive tract and metabolism. This incomplete burning of fat produces acetic acid.

## Refined Foods

White sugar and white flour products, candy, soft drinks, many drugs and processed foods are all acid-forming foods. This is because they are lacking in minerals and must rob minerals from the body tissues in order to be metabolized.

As little as two teaspoons of refined white sugar is enough to change mineral relationships in the body. All minerals work in relation to one another, so changing those relationships means some minerals will be unavailable when needed.

Researchers have found that eating sugar increases the excretion of calcium in the urine. This alone can upset the mineral balance in the body. When sugar is eaten day after day and year after year, it stresses the balance or homeostasis of the body.

Other studies have shown that two teaspoons of sugar is enough to significantly decrease the number of white blood cells, leading to immune system suppression.

## Alkaline- and Acid-Forming Foods

Foods are determined to be acid- or alkaline-forming according to the residue or ash they leave in the body. In the following list of common foods, notice that alkaline ash comes primarily from fruits and vegetables and acid ash comes primarily from meats, grains and refined carbohydrates. There is often confusion about acidic fruits such as lemons, oranges and grapefruit. These fruits have an alkalizing effect on the body because their acids are "burned" by the body, giving off carbon dioxide and water and leaving an alkaline mineral ash.

| **Alkaline-Forming Foods:** | **Acid-Forming Foods:** |
| --- | --- |
| almonds | bread |
| apple | cake |
| apricot | cereals (processed) |
| artichoke | cornflakes |
| avocado | crackers |
| banana | cranberry |
| beans: | dairy products |
|    most dried beans | eggs |
|    lima | fish: |
|    navy |    codfish |
|    snap |    haddock |
| beets and beet greens |    salmon |
| berries: |    sardines |
|    blackberry |    tuna |
|    blueberry | flours: |
|    gooseberry |    whole wheat |
|    raspberry |    white flour |

## Alkaline-Forming Foods:

strawberry
broccoli
brussels sprouts
buckwheat
cabbage
carrots
cauliflower
celery
chard, Swiss
cherry
chestnuts
chives
coconut
cucumber
currants
dandelion greens
dates
eggplant
endive
garlic
grapefruit
grapes
figs
kale
kohlrabi
lemon
lettuce
lime
mango
melons:
  cantaloupe
  watermelon
millet
molasses
mushrooms

## Acid-Forming Foods:

grains:
  barley
  oats
  rye
  wheat
  corn
macaroni
mayonnaise
meats:
  bacon
  beef
  chicken
  corned beef
  duck
  ham
  lamb
  liver
  pork
  sausage
  turkey
  veal
muffins
nuts
oatmeal
pastries
peanuts
peanut butter
pies
plum
prunes
rice:
  brown rice
  white rice
shellfish:
  clams

**Alkaline-Forming Foods:**
nectarine
okra
olives
onion
orange
parsley
peach
peas
pear
peppers
pineapple
potato
pumpkin
radish
raisins
rhubarb
rutabaga
spinach
sprouts
squash
tangerine
tomato
turnip and turnip greens
watercress
yam

**Acid-Forming Foods:**
crab
shrimp
lobster
oysters
scallops
lentils
persimmon
soybeans
spaghetti
wheat germ

**Neutral with Acidifying Effect:**
fats
olive oil
sugar syrups
sugar, refined
   (white and brown)

## Your Cells in Allergy

Cells require specific conditions in order to stay healthy. If a cell's environment changes sufficiently and exceeds its capacity to maintain normal homeostasis or balance, we get acute cell injury. If enough cells are injured, pathology results. It is said that we live or die at the cellular level. What conditions are necessary for cells to live in a healthy state?

An important condition is maintenance of the optimum pH of cells. Cellular enzymes, which control all functions of the cell, require a very narrow pH range. If the pH of the cell becomes too acid or alkaline, enzymatic function decreases and impairs survival of the cell. The pH also affects the function of insulin. Insulin moves glucose (a form of sugar) through the cell membrane to be burned for energy. If the extra-cellular fluids are not alkaline enough, glucose cannot enter the cell. The result is fatigue.

Cells must have a constant oxygen supply. When glucose enters the cell, it combines with oxygen in tiny organelles called mitochondria to produce ATP (adenosine triphosphate). ATP is the energy reserve or stored energy. When sufficient oxygen is available, between 32 and 36 moles of ATP per glucose unit are produced. If insufficient oxygen is supplied, as few as 3 moles of ATP per unit of glucose are produced. This is a considerable difference in ATP production, representing a much lowered energy production.

Research indicates that blood can carry the maximum amount of oxygen to your cells at the specific pH of 7.4. Therefore, any degree of acidosis or alkalosis would decrease the oxygen-carrying capacity of the blood and decrease energy production.

Diet is the greatest single stimulus affecting the blood, because eating is something that happens every day, several times a day. Two to five pounds of food are metabolized daily. For the average person, two-thirds of the calories in the diet are from fat and sugar. When acid metabolites are produced faster than they can be neutralized, the blood pH changes and symptoms develop. Over-consumption of fats leads to acidosis by impeding the supply of nutrients and oxygen to the cells.

Minerals are also required for cells to function properly, and they must be balanced in proportion to one another. Sodium is found primarily in the fluids *surrounding* the cell while potassium is found primarily in the fluids *inside* the cell. If sodium decreases, fluid will flow into the cell, impeding cellular function. If sodium increases outside the cell, the fluid will flow from the cell to the surrounding tissue. Too much or not enough – both situations are undesirable. Balance is what is required.

What happens when an allergic reaction takes place in the tissues? How do cells react? Let's first look at the life of a normal cell.

We have in our bodies an estimated 70 to 100 trillion cells, each one like a little factory. Each cell is an expert in the processes of manufacturing, transportation and waste disposal. The cell depends on the blood stream and the extra-cellular fluids to bring it raw materials. It depends on the same fluids to carry away the waste. If the waste is not carried away quickly, its toxicity can damage the cell. If the proper raw materials are not supplied, cellular function can be compromised and damage can occur.

What kind of factory is the cell? It is an energy producer. For the cell to survive and thrive, it must be able to generate enough energy to grow, to repair itself, to reproduce and to do the special work of the tissue it comprises. Oxygen, nutrients and intracellular enzymes are necessary for the cell to generate energy. Anything that compromises these three essentials threatens the survival of the cell. In addition, elimination of waste is essential. No cell can survive surrounded by its own refuse. The fluid surrounding the cell must remain clean, of proper mineral balance, of sufficient quantity and of constant pH.

Therefore, a proper nutrient supply linked with proper waste disposal and proper environment is the only way that the health of the cell can be maintained. If all of the cells are healthy there can be no allergy or any other disease in the body!

Likewise, the body as a whole has the same requirements as each cell. It must have oxygen and nutrients in order for it to grow, repair itself, reproduce and fulfill its function in the world. It must have an efficiently working waste disposal system (bowels, kidneys, lungs, skin). This is the only way that health can be maintained.

What happens to the cell when these conditions are not met? What happens to the cell when it encounters allergy?

When an allergic reaction takes place, the cells involved release toxic products of allergic inflammation, which can penetrate the cell membranes of surrounding cells and cause the capillaries to become leaky.

In the cells directly affected by allergic swelling, allergic inflammation manifests itself. It is the lysosome, the digestive organelle inside the cell, which swells. The membrane of the lysosome is disrupted, causing hydrolytic enzymes to pour out and destroy the

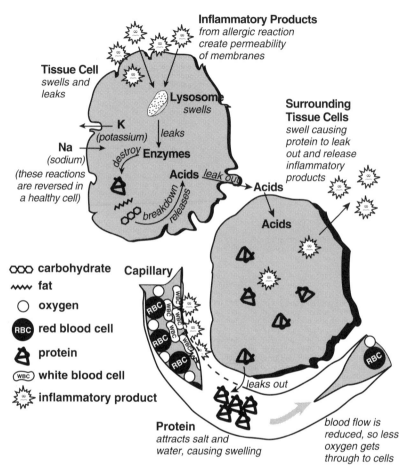

**Inflammatory Products**
*from allergic reaction
create permeability
of membranes*

**Tissue Cell**
*swells and
leaks*

**Lysosome**
*swells*

K
*(potassium)*

*leaks*

**Na**
*(sodium)*

*destroy* **Enzymes**

*(these reactions
are reversed in
a healthy cell)*

*breakdown*

*releases*

**Acids** *leak out*

**Surrounding
Tissue Cells**
*swell causing
protein to leak
out and release
inflammatory
products*

➤**Acids**

**Acids**

∞ **carbohydrate**

∿ **fat**

○ **oxygen**

(RBC) **red blood cell**

▲ **protein**

(WBC) **white blood cell**

✸ **inflammatory product**

**Capillary**

*leaks out*

**Protein**
*attracts salt and
water, causing swelling*

*blood flow is
reduced, so less
oxygen gets
through to cells*

*Figure 3.* **The Cell Encounters Allergy**

protein, carbohydrate and fat within the cell. This creates acids which cause an acid pH inside the cell. We all know what acid rain does to our lakes. When an allergic reaction takes place, it is the equivalent of acid rain in the cells. The cell membrane leaks these acids into the fluids surrounding the cell. Potassium inside the cell is lost to the outside of the cell and sodium enters the cell, causing more swelling or edema.

As the body continues to respond to the allergic injury, protein leaks out of surrounding cells due to inflammatory toxins which have caused capillary permeability (leakiness). The proteins coagulate outside the capillaries, causing the red blood cells to sludge, or slow down and stick together. The white blood cells stick to the capillary walls trying to plug the leaks. The result is that oxygen is inhibited from reaching the involved cells and acid waste products accumulate.

Lack of oxygen, slowed blood flow and increased acidity in the tissues together cause changes in the cell metabolism and lactic acid begins to build up, increasing acidity. The changes in cell metabolism can be mild to severe and they can be local or widespread. When enough tissue changes have occurred, symptoms develop. These can range all the way from slight fatigue to incapacitating illness, depending on the location and extensiveness of the injury.

# 10

# Digestion – The Vital Link

If you eat an average North American diet, you are virtually guaranteed to develop a chronic degenerative disease at some point in your lifetime. This can be illustrated by the ten major diseases which afflict an estimated 100 million Americans. These diseases are:

| | | |
|---|---|---|
| heart disease | obesity | alcoholism |
| cancer | diabetes | addiction |
| stroke | arthritis | mental illness |
| high blood pressure | | |

Of the above ten diseases, eight have been established as being diet related and the other two have known dietary components. *The Kellogg Report* of May, 1990 by Joseph D. Beasley, MD and Jerry Swift, MA, explores the impact of nutrition, environment and lifestyle on the health of Americans. It reports, "Perhaps the clearest concrete example of the effects of nutritional inadequacy can be found in the elderly: one of the most basic reasons they catch pneumonia or break bones at far higher rates than others (and than they themselves did when younger) is that their resistance and resilience have long been undermined by inadequate nutrition. As we grow older we need fewer and fewer calories but just as many or more nutrients each day. Thus, we all require an increasingly nutrient-dense diet as the years pass, a need that is scarcely recognized and rarely met in contemporary America."

*No race in history has ever attempted to live on the diet that North Americans are now eating.* There is no scientific proof that we can healthfully live on it. There is now appearing considerable evidence that we cannot. More and more authorities are becoming aware that adequate diet is an absolutely necessary pre-condition to a healthy life.

In the United States, one out of three surgeries takes place because of digestive problems. One in ten deaths is attributed to digestive disorders. The vast majority of digestive conditions develop slowly over a long period of time. Many people think that if they do not have pain or discomfort in their stomachs, they do not have digestive disorders. Excessive gas, belching, burning, diarrhea and constipation are all symptoms signaling that the digestive process is not proceeding normally and should not be ignored.

Allergy can be characterized as a chronic degenerative disease which is diet-related, and is affecting more people today than ever before. Let's explore why.

Eating a diet high in fat, sugar and refined, processed foods alters normal digestion. Digestion is the cornerstone of nutrition. It is also a cornerstone to understanding allergy. When you eat food, it goes through a series of chemical breakdowns called digestion. Proteins break down into amino acids, carbohydrates break down into glucose and fats break down into fatty acids. When this breaking down fails to happen, symptoms occur. When foods are fully digested, they enter the blood stream in the normal way. The body recognizes them as nutrients and utilizes them accordingly. If they are not in the correct form when they enter the blood stream, the body recognizes them as foreign invaders and attacks as if they were viruses or bacteria.

The most common food allergens are milk, egg, wheat, nuts, corn, soy and beef. All of these foods in various breakdown stages yield protein products. It is no coincidence that most food allergens are protein fragments from poorly digested meat, dairy products and the protein portion of wheat. Most bacteria and foreign invaders are also protein in nature, so the body is already programmed to attack unidentifiable protein particles. When the food is fully digested into its proper end products, it has lost its ability to be allergenic. In the textbook *Human Nutrition* we find that "Any major alteration of the molecular structure usually results in loss of allergic potential, thus digestion with the attendant splitting of the molecules into peptides and amino acids renders the protein non-allergic, depending on the extent of the hydrolytic degradation."

Traditional medical treatment considers abstinence from the food allergen to be the most effective treatment. While this may relieve symptoms, it will not get the person well. Avoiding the food is treating the symptom rather than the cause. The egg is not the cause of the patient's symptoms, although the egg may very well induce all kinds of reactions. Helping an incompetent digestive tract to work better is a more rational approach. It is necessary to eliminate the egg only until the digestive tract is healed and functioning normally. If you can't digest the egg, you can't get its nutrients, but you can get allergic reactions.

Amino acids are the end products of protein digestion. It is the amino acid which is absorbed from the intestine and circulated in the blood to the cells. The cells are extremely creative with these amino acids. They link them together in chain-like structures, to make new proteins capable of specific functions. Proteins make up about three-fourths of the solid portions of the body. Each cell is a mixture of proteins and a single cell can contain hundreds of combinations of proteins.

In the lottery game 6/49, six numbers are picked from a possible 49 numbers. We are told there are approximately 14 million combinations possible from these 49 numbers. We know that there are about 20 major amino acids in the body and thousands of lesser-known amino acids. Even with just the 20 amino acids, we have the possibility of more than seven million combinations if they were linked six at a time. However, the average number of amino acids linked together in the body is 400 and even the smallest protein has 20 amino acids, not six. The actual number of combinations possible is estimated to be infinite. Given this information, will we ever have complete control over even this one body process? It is unlikely. The control which we have is in our ability to choose what stimulus we give our body, positive or negative. We must give our body what it needs to do the work it has to do. Then let the body do its job. If one farmer is given a shovel and another farmer is given a tractor, which farmer will be able to do the most work? The control you have remains with the lifestyle choices you make as to what you eat, drink, think and expose your body to.

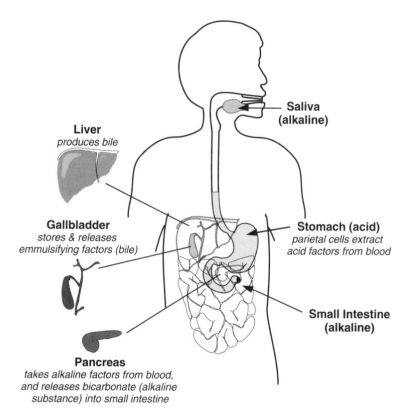

*Figure 4.* **Alkaline and Acid Organs of Digestion**

Digestion begins when you chew your food. Saliva enzymes coat the food before it is swallowed, going through the esophagus to the stomach. In the stomach, enzymes continue to break down the food for up to an hour before the stomach becomes too acid for the enzymes to work. Enzyme activity is dependent upon the pH. Each enzyme works within a very specific pH range. The enzymes from the saliva work in an alkaline solution, and hence are inactivated in an acid stomach environment. However, other enzymes now go to work. The stomach's hydrochloric acid converts pepsinogen to pepsin, an active proteolytic enzyme. The acid mulch produced in the stomach is slowly passed or squeezed through the pyloric valve into the small intestine where it encounters an alkaline environment, created by the bicarbonate from the pancreas. The acid stomach enzymes are now inactivated by the alkalinity, but the saliva enzymes may be reactivated. The pancreas has also supplied additional enzymes to work in this final digestive process. Protein-, carbohydrate- and fat-digesting enzymes are all supplied on demand by the pancreas.

However, the raw materials for all these enzymes must be supplied from the blood. If the raw materials are not in the blood in sufficient quantities, digestion will not take place normally. Abnormal digestion may not necessarily produce pain, so the person may not know when digestion is no longer competent. If pain is produced, however, it is a major warning flag. If a person seeks medical help at this time, often no tissue changes have taken place that can be diagnosed as a disease. Therefore, no help is forthcoming. After months or years of incompetent digestion and ever-increasing symptomatology, recognizable tissue changes will result, and the diagnosis of disease is finally made.

Somewhere in between, allergies often develop, because any time there is tissue injury in the digestive tract, large, undigested food particles have the opportunity to enter the blood stream. The resultant attack on them by the immune system creates the allergic reaction.

The vital function of digestion is totally dependent upon the pH of the blood, and the pH of the blood is dependent primarily upon the food that you eat. The reason that digestion is dependent upon the pH of the blood is that the acid-forming elements, hydrogen and chloride, must be present in the blood in sufficient quantities for the stomach's parietal cells to place the end product of hydrochloric acid in the stomach. Parietal cells must get their raw materials from somewhere, and in this case, it is from the blood stream. Parietal cells communicate with the blood through a system of intracellular caniculi. If the blood has too much alkalinity, hydrochloric acid formation in the stomach is diminished, because the blood will not release its acid substances.

One common source of excess alkalinity is the constant taking of drugs such as antacids. Antacids flood the blood stream as well as the stomach with alkalinity. This neutralizes the hydrogen in the blood and makes it unavailable to the parietal cells to form hydrochloric acid. If hydrochloric acid cannot be formed, the stomach enzymes pepsinogen and pepsin cannot work, as they require an acid pH of around 2 to 3. Since pepsin works on protein, protein digestion in the stomach cannot take place efficiently.

A similar situation occurs in the small intestine. When the acidic stomach contents enter the small intestine, the pH of the small intestine falls below 4.0, which is acid. However, digestion here requires an alkaline pH. The acidity triggers an enzyme called secretin to be released in large quantities, stimulating the immediate release of bicarbonate which is very alkaline. The alkaline bicarbonate is formed in the ductile cells of the pancreas from substances extracted from the blood. If the concentration of these substances is below their respective thresholds, they will remain in the blood and not be available for the purpose of digestion. This is because maintenance of blood pH gets first priority for survival. Only when a sufficient quantity of materials is present in the blood can they be released for digestive purposes.

Drugs often interfere with the intricate digestive process. For example, the drug acetazolamide is commonly used for glaucoma and altitude sickness. By inhibiting an important enzyme, this drug almost completely blocks the formation of hydrochloric acid. This, of course, interferes with digestion.

## Microflora of the Intestines

Besides faulty digestion, another condition is often involved in allergy. Originally known as "intestinal toxemia," this condition has recently gained new acceptance under the name of "enterotoxemia." Enterotoxemia simply means a condition characterized by presence in the blood of toxins produced in the intestines. The microflora, organisms which live in the intestines, play a role. Exactly what the role of the microflora is has been controversial in scientific circles since the turn of the century, with some doctors lending it great importance and others dismissing it outright.

While much information has yet to be discovered about enterotoxemia, there are some well established facts.

1. There are over four hundred species of microorganisms present in the normal intestines.

2. These normal microorganisms participate in many functions important to the health of the body. They help balance blood cholesterol levels and hormone levels, support immune function, participate in the production of some nutrients, and suppress the growth of pathogenic organisms.

3. The type and quantity of these beneficial organisms are directly affected by the diet. The food eaten is also food for the bacteria. The more a certain type of food is eaten, the more the bacteria specific to it can grow. For example, when a high protein diet is eaten, proteolytic bacteria proliferate in the intestine.

4. Many toxic products of bacterial decomposition are absorbed from the intestine into the blood stream. These products are conveyed to the liver for detoxification. The fact that toxins are absorbed from the intestine is evidenced in many laboratory studies.

Indole is formed from tryptophan, an amino acid derived from protein and delivered to the liver for detoxification. This is the basis for the common urine indican test as a measure of protein digestion.

However, what if the toxin is present in too large a quantity for the liver to detoxify? What if there are toxins that the liver cannot detoxify?

Phenol is an example of a toxin produced in the bowel from the amino acid tyrosine in the process of putrefaction. Most of the phenol is not detoxified by the liver. Phenol – the product of incomplete protein digestion – has the ability to kill cells, especially liver and kidney cells. The presence in the blood of toxic products of decomposition can be increased by any defect of the intestinal lining.

Permeability of the intestinal lining can have a number of causes. A prestigious medical journal, *The Lancet* (Saturday, 28 January,

1984, "The Leaky Gut of Alcoholism") reported that alcohol drinkers who abstained from alcohol for four days still had greater intestinal permeability than a non-drinking control group. For many, the abnormality persisted for up to two weeks after they stopped drinking.

Anti-inflammatory drugs affect intestinal permeability, as described in *The Lancet* (Saturday, 24 November, 1984, "Intestinal Permeability and Inflammation in Rheumatoid Arthritis"). Intestinal permeability was almost invariably abnormal in patients treated with non-steroidal anti-inflammatory drugs.

Numerous toxins are produced in the colon, especially where there is alteration of the ratio of normal flora to pathogenic flora. Increased numbers of pathogenic organisms can produce pathogenic substances. For example, Candida and other yeasts ferment dietary sugars to ethyl alcohol and acetylaldehyde. They also increase the permeability of the intestine, allowing their toxic products to enter the blood stream.

Ammonia is another substance produced in the intestine by bacterial action on proteins. If this ammonia enters the blood stream, known neurological symptoms develop, such as confusion, drowsiness, mental disturbances, tremors and altered EEG patterns. Ammonia is normally converted in the liver to urea. However, when the amount of ammonia overwhelms the liver's capacity to convert the ammonia, neurological symptoms have been observed.

Many toxins produced by microflora have not been studied in great detail, but the few that have been studied should alert us to the importance of maintaining healthy flora in the intestines.

Some symptoms that have been linked to improper gut flora include:

| | | |
|---|---|---|
| allergy | fatigue | sinusitis |
| nervousness | rashes | heartbeat irregularities |
| acne | arthritis | hormonal disturbances |
| headaches | asthma | ear inflammation |
| low back pain | intestinal symptoms | |

The diet producing the lowest levels of toxins, and thus considered to be the most efficient in lowering toxin production and

increasing nutrient values is:
1. A low protein, high complex carbohydrate diet with abundant fresh fruits and vegetables.
2. A diet in which small to moderate amounts of food are eaten. All food, if eaten in too great a quantity for the digestive enzymes to process, can lead to the production of toxins.

Two excerpts from articles linking the ecology of the bowel microflora to allergy are provided below.

Hugh A Sampson, MD, in the *Journal of the American College of Nutrition* (Volume 9, #4, 1990), states that, "The development of food allergy is the result of an interaction between food allergens, the gastrointestinal tract and the immune system."

"Intestinal Permeability, Acquired CHO Intolerance," published by John Hopkins University Press 1981, states that, "It has long been known that macromolecular permeability might be altered in gastroenteritis since there is measurable absorption of egg albumin and there are frequently milk protein antibodies present in serum following diarrhea. Increased macromolecular absorption may lead to the development of hypersensitivity and allergy to foodstuffs in the susceptible host."

# 11

# The Enzyme Answer to Allergy

Presenting enzyme therapy as the key to healing allergies makes this book unique. Enzyme therapy has long been the missing chapter in other allergy books. Yet enzyme therapy is so powerful that it renders the common or traditional therapies for allergy unnecessary. Following enzyme therapy, a person can often add back to his diet the foods to which he was once allergic rather than avoiding these foods for life. Constant elimination and rotation of foods is not required. Understanding enzyme therapy and the role of digestion is the first giant step to overcoming allergic conditions.

"Enzymes are substances that make life possible. They are needed for every chemical reaction that takes place in the human body. No mineral, vitamin, or hormone can do any work without enzymes." This quote is from the book *Enzyme Nutrition* by Dr. Edward Howell. Enzymes sound important, but what are they? And how are they related to allergy? To know the answer to this last question is to understand what the vast majority of doctors and health professionals have failed to realize. Yet the necessary information is well documented. It is sitting, for the most part, unused in medical libraries around North America.

Let's start at the beginning. For years scientists have considered enzymes to be organic compounds capable of accelerating or producing some change in (by breaking down) a substance for which they are usually specific. However, Dr. Howell considers enzymes specialized "protein carriers charged with vital energy factors." He likens them to the battery of a flashlight. When the battery has energy, the flashlight lights up. When the battery is dead, it will not activate the flashlight. However, the battery itself looks the same in both cases. Dr. Howell believes enzymes work the same way. An example is two seeds. The first seed is planted in the soil. The second seed is boiled first and then planted. Only the first seed will grow because it contains live enzymes, although both seeds look the same. The growing seed is an example of enzyme activity. Other examples of enzyme activity are ripening of fruit and leaves changing color in the fall. In the human body, absolutely every activity requires enzymes: eating, breathing, sleeping, working and even thinking.

The amino acids derived from protein have long been considered to be the building blocks of the cell. However, the enzymes are the workers that put the amino acids together. This is the difference between having a pile of bricks and having a brick house. The bricks (amino acids) cannot be put together without workers (enzymes). Every activity of the body is dependent upon enzymes. Enzymes digest food, activate the immune system and build minerals into bone. Male sperm carries enzymes that dissolve part of the female egg membrane in order for the sperm to gain entrance to the ovum and fertilize it.

Each organ and tissue has its own specialized enzymes to do the work required. Ninety-eight different enzymes have been found in the arteries alone, helping to keep them clean and functional. In fact, a whole book on just the enzymes in the arteries has been written. About 5,000 individual enzymes have so far been isolated and identified, but some authorities estimate that it takes about 100,000 enzymes to run the body, each with a specific job to do.

Is it possible to have an enzyme deficiency? The answer is yes and that is why it is important to know about enzymes. Even though there are thousands of different enzymes, there are basically only three types: digestive enzymes that digest food, metabolic enzymes that run the body and food enzymes that are found in raw food.

Of these, the digestive enzymes, protease, lipase and amylase are the most well known. Protease breaks protein down into amino acids, lipase breaks fat down into fatty acids and amylase breaks starch down into glucose. Enzymes are very specific in their function. For example, protease can only digest protein; it cannot break down fat. Likewise, lipase digests only fat, not protein.

Enzymes have specific acid/alkaline ranges they work in. The enzyme chymotrypsin can only work in a very alkaline range, while pepsin must have a very acid environment. If pepsin is put in an alkaline solution, it is inactivated. Enzymes also have their own particular temperature range. They are inactive outside that range. A pear will ripen at room temperature faster than a pear put in the refrigerator, because the pear at room temperature will have more enzyme activity.

Enzymes are the key to understanding allergy. Years ago, one author stated that 90 percent of all food allergy could be eliminated if people chewed their food well. The book did not explain why, probably because the author did not know, but may have noticed a relationship. Now, of course, we know why this is good advice. When food is chewed well, it is thoroughly mixed with enzymes from the saliva. Enzymes work on the surfaces of the food particles which means that the more thoroughly chewed the food is, the more exposed surfaces there are for enzymes to work on. Also, the cells of fruits and vegetables have indigestible cellulose membranes which must be broken down by chewing before the fruit or vegetable can be digested. Many adverse reactions to fresh produce result simply from not chewing sufficiently to break down the cellulose membranes.

The teeth are very efficient if allowed to do their work. Using the jaw muscles, studies show that the front teeth (incisors) can close with a force of up to 55 pounds. The back teeth (molars) can close with a force of up to 200 pounds. With a small piece of food between the molars, the actual force per square inch can be up to several thousand pounds.

Many nutritionists advise chewing each bite twenty to fifty times. For the allergic person, chewing each bite to liquid is better advice. Once the habit of chewing thoroughly is established, it does not require much conscious thought.

When a banana is eaten, it is first chewed in the mouth. The chewing action breaks the cell walls of the banana, liberating the enzymes stored in the banana. These enzymes immediately start to digest the banana. The banana is mixed with saliva in the mouth, which helps to activate the food enzymes in the banana. Saliva itself contains three kinds of enzymes from three sets of glands in the mouth. However, since the banana supplies its own enzymes, not many enzymes from the salivary glands are required and the glands respond accordingly with less production. All these enzymes work well in an alkaline mouth pH.

The macerated banana proceeds to the stomach. Distension of the stomach along with enzyme action signals for hydrochloric acid production to take place. It takes 45 minutes to one hour for sufficient hydrochloric acid to build up in the stomach to inactivate the alkaline enzymes. During this time up to 60 percent of the starch, 30 percent of the protein and 10 percent of the fat of a food can be digested. In fact, studies done at the University of Illinois have demonstrated that up to 80 percent of the carbohydrates are digested during this time by saliva enzymes only. And this is before the stomach begins digestion! In other words, by eating raw foods and chewing them well, a major portion of digestion will take place before the stomach does any work. Since this example is a raw banana, which is mostly carbohydrate and low in protein and fat, there is not much stimulus for the stomach to secrete a great deal of hydrochloric acid or enzymes. The banana now moves on through the pyloric valve to the small intestine. Here it encounters an alkaline environment again, since the pancreas is supplying alkaline bicarbonate. Some of the banana enzymes and the saliva enzymes that were inactivated by the acid stomach pH can again go to work in this alkaline environment. The pancreas will supply any additional enzymes necessary to complete the task. Again, in this case, not many enzymes are needed. The digested banana now is broken down into a form ready to be absorbed through the intestinal membranes and into the blood stream. This is the normal sequence of events. The digestive organs were able to work normally with no particular stress placed upon them.

But what happens if you consume a piece of fried chicken instead? The chicken contains no enzymes of its own because it has been cooked at temperatures above 118°F (48°C), the temperature at which enzymes are destroyed. Let's say that it is gulped down in chunks rather than chewed thoroughly. Because it was not chewed well, it reaches the stomach with little enzyme activity from the saliva and none from the chicken itself. The stomach has a lot more work to do in this case, as the chicken can sit in the stomach for the first hour with little digestion taking place. After the enzymes build up in the stomach, they digest some of the chicken and it eventually moves on to the small intestine. Here, bile from the gall bladder enters and emulsifies the fat of the chicken. However, bile contains no enzymes. That leaves the remainder of the work to the pancreas, which must now call in all of its resources to supply digestive enzymes to complete the digestion. This places an extra burden on the pancreas.

Studies show that when the diet consists of mostly cooked foods containing no enzymes, the pancreas will actually enlarge to keep up with the demand. This is called pancreatic hypertrophy. The significance of this is that the types of food eaten affect the health of the pancreas. When the pancreas must produce greater amounts of enzymes than normal, it enlarges. The same thing happens to your heart if it must pump blood through arteries that are clogged with cholesterol. Enlargement of an organ has long been associated with pathology. When laboratory mice are fed heat-treated or cooked food with no enzymes, their pancreases weigh two to three times as much as those of wild mice eating raw food.

The consequences of excess demand on the pancreas are described in the book *Victory over Diabetes,* by William H. Philpott, MD and Dwight K. Kalita, PhD: "An over stimulated pancreas follows the same general law that other over stimulated tissues and organ systems follow, namely, that over stimulation eventually leads to inhibition of function. It is well documented that addiction to alcohol leads to pancreatic insufficiency. What has been little appreciated in the past is that all addictions, be they food, chemical, or otherwise lead to pancreatic insufficiency in varying degrees." Dr. Philpott goes on to say that the pancreas is the first endocrine/exocrine organ to come in contact with ingested foods or chemicals, and as such is a common shock organ for those foods or chemicals. Remember, the shock organ is the place where the cells release their toxic products during an allergic reaction.

A human weighing 140 pounds has a pancreas weighing approximately 85-95 grams. The pancreas of a sheep weighing 84 pounds is only 19 grams. If the sheep doubled its weight to 170 pounds its pancreas would still weigh only 38 grams, or less than half the weight of a human pancreas. The sheep eats all raw food – a high enzyme diet, needing less help from the pancreas.

The pancreas works according to the law of adaptive secretion. This means that enzymes are secreted by the pancreas on demand. The quantity and type of food determines the quantity and type of enzymes secreted. For example, a large, starchy meal of pasta will stimulate large amounts of amylase, whereas a steak will cause an abundance of protease to be secreted. In other words, there is specific secretion for specific foods. The pancreas will secrete only the types and amounts of enzymes it needs for the job at hand. It will not secrete more than necessary. However, when highly refined, cooked food is eaten, the food contributes no enzymes and the demand on the pancreas goes up. In 1943, Northwestern University established the law of adaptive secretion by experiments on rats. The amount of digestive enzymes secreted by the pancreas in response to carbohydrate, protein and fat was measured, and it was found that the quantity of each enzyme varied with the amount of the food it was to digest.

Besides enlargement, another condition results when cooked foods with no enzymes are ingested. The condition, called digestive leukocytosis, is an increase of white blood cells in the blood stream. Leukocytosis, generally considered a pathological condition, can be observed in cases of infection, intoxication and poisoning. In 1930 Paul Kautchakoff, MD proved that leukocytosis can also be caused by ingesting cooked food. His findings were as follows: raw or frozen foods caused no leukocytosis; common cooked foods caused a mild leukocytosis; pressure-cooked and canned foods caused a moderate leukocytosis; processed or highly refined foods (such as carbonated beverages, alcohol, vinegar, white sugar and white flour products) caused severe leukocytosis. Canned meat was the worst, bringing on a violent reaction equivalent to what might be seen in poisoning.

Why is this leukocytosis happening? We know that white blood cells are the ones that defend us against invading organisms. The white blood cells carry many enzymes. It is the enzyme activity that allows the white blood cell to engulf and destroy bacteria and viruses. The pancreas is a small organ, even in the enlarged state, and cannot itself produce all of the enzymes necessary to digest the food eaten, since that food averages up to five pounds a day. The pancreas gets its raw materials from the blood stream. It can secrete and store a limited amount of enzymes. When the pancreas is over-stressed and over-stimulated, the white blood cells, or leukocytes, which have ample supplies of enzymes, are transported to the digestive tract to aid in the digestive process. This is a compensatory mechanism of the body in times of undue stress. Cooked food contains no enzymes, but the pancreas requires those missing food enzymes in conjunction with its stored digestive enzymes to digest food. When food enzymes are not present, the pancreas must call in the reserves – the white blood cells.

Enzymes are produced by all cells of the body. After a raw food meal there is no increase in the number of white blood cells in the blood stream. When cooked food is eaten, the whole body has to work much harder to produce and transport enzymes for the job of digestion. This leaves fewer enzymes to do metabolic work for the rest of the body. In nature, the pancreas was never intended to secrete 100 percent of the enzymes needed each time food is eaten.

What does this have to do with the immune system? *Here is the vital link.* If leukocytes are giving up their enzymes to aid in the digestive process, they will have fewer enzymes for destroying bacteria and foreign invaders. With fewer enzymes, the leukocytes become sluggish and immobile. This is the mechanism by which you can impair your immune system every time you eat. The body's immune response is being mobilized to compensate for a lack of enzymes in the food. This can exhaust your immune system needlessly. There is a connection between the strength of the immune system and the body's enzyme levels. The greater the level of enzymes, the stronger the immune system and the healthier the person.

Enzymes can and do become depleted. Meyer and his associates at Michael Resse Hospital, Chicago, performed an experiment on the amylase of saliva. Two groups of subjects were used. In one group, the average age was 25 years and in another group the average age was 81 years. The amylase content in the saliva was 30 times greater in the younger group. These investigators found that young people can easily digest 50 grams of white bread in the mouth and stomach, while only one percent of it will be digested in the mouth and stomach of the older people. In general, high enzyme values are found in the tissues of young people and low values are found in older individuals with exhausted tissues. It is interesting to note that the enzyme content of body fluids is also low in chronic degenerative diseases, indicating tissue enzyme depletion.

It is estimated that 20 million Americans have various digestive disorders. Sales of the stomach medication Tagamet have topped even the sales of Valium in recent years. Digestive difficulties are also apparent from the billions of dollars spent on over-the-counter antacids and laxatives. The following are some of the symptoms of pancreatic enzyme deficiency: gas after meals, bloating of the abdomen, skin problems, recurring headaches, muscle wasting and depression.

According to Dr. Philpott, when the pancreas is over-stimulated, the bicarbonate production is the first function to be inhibited. This is a function not given its proper place of importance, for it plays a major role in the acid-base balance of the body. Without sufficient bicarbonate production, the acid from the stomach cannot be adequately neutralized in the small intestine and the whole body can become acidic. The second function to suffer in pancreatic insufficiency is enzyme production. The consequence here, of course, is compromised digestion, particularly of protein. When protein cannot be broken down into amino acids, new enzymes cannot be built, as amino acids are the raw material required for enzyme production. Enzymes are protein compounds made from various combinations of amino acids. The body requires amino acids since approximately three-fourths of the solid parts of the body are protein, all built from amino acids.

The last function to be compromised in an over-taxed pancreas is insulin production. Insulin is best known as the substance needed by diabetics, but there is another aspect to diabetes. Diabetics also have been shown to have lowered blood levels of the enzyme amylase. The essential thing to remember is that the pancreas cannot be over-taxed without stressing the whole body.

Some enzyme deficiencies are well documented, such as lactase deficiency. When this enzyme is deficient, a person can experience gas, bloating, diarrhea, gastritis and pain from drinking milk simply because that one enzyme is lacking. When the enzyme phenylalanine hydroxylase is absent in babies, phenylalanine accumulates in the tissues and can kill or mentally retard the baby unless it is treated. This condition is called phenylketonuria or PKU. Dr. Jonathan Brostoff reports on an experiment done on chemical- and food-sensitive individuals in *The Complete Guide to Food Allergy and Intolerance*. In the group which was sensitive to chemicals, 90 percent were deficient for one enzyme. In the food intolerant group, 80 percent were deficient for one enzyme.

These are only some examples of enzyme deficiency and its consequences. Many enzyme deficiencies remain "hidden," producing slow, less severe symptoms and are difficult to confirm. Even so, numerous clinical studies have demonstrated that enzyme deficiencies do occur in allergic, chemical-sensitive and food intolerant individuals.

### CASE STUDY: *Mary*

Mary, age 33, arrived at my office with a history of mental confusion, depression, suicidal tendencies, hyperactivity and inability to cope as a housewife and mother to three small children. She had been in and out of mental hospitals many times over the years. Examination revealed many digestive symptoms, and intolerance of yeast and nuts. She was also deficient in vitamin A. Additional foods and environmental allergies were suspected. Treatment consisted of enzyme therapy, a program for candidiasis, multiple minerals, a nutritional thyroid formula, a B-complex formula and vitamins A, C and E. Body organs were strengthened with specific reflex adjustments along the spine.

Because of her mental condition, this patient was unable to follow a treatment program consistently. Results were proportional to her compliance to the program. For example, Mary tested allergic to smoke but did not stop smoking. However, she did manage to follow the instructions enough to notice improvement. Although she was up and down a lot mentally, she recognized that she was getting better. Enzyme therapy seemed to particularly benefit her, as it appeared to halt the many reactions to foods and other substances

Since her treatment, Mary no longer has the suicidal tendencies or severe depression. Her general health has improved along with her digestion. She no longer requires hospitalization. All symptoms have cleared except for mild episodes of hyperactivity and some mental "fog." This patient appears to be a fairly good example of the effects on the brain of food and environmental chemicals. Outlook for this patient is good if she continues to work to eliminate additional stressors to the body such as tobacco smoke, and if she continues her nutritional and enzyme therapy.

The concept of multiple enzyme deficiency has never been explored. In cases of allergy, multiple enzyme deficiencies appear to prevail.

One way we know that low serum levels of enzymes induce allergy is through the research of Dr. Oelgoetz, an MD who performed experiments in the 1930s. When doses of pancreatic enzymes were given to patients with allergic symptoms and low serum enzyme levels, the serum enzyme levels returned to normal and the allergy subsided. Dr. Oelgoetz believed that when large, undigested food molecules enter the blood stream, the enzymes in the blood complete the process of digestion of the partially digested material. A low level of serum enzymes cannot do this.

Studies done by the Potter Metabolic Clinic in Santa Barbara, California showed good results in allergic disorders with the administration of enzymes. These results found bronchial asthma 88 percent improved, asthma induced by food 92 percent improved and eczema from food 83 percent improved.

## CASE STUDY: *Ray*

Violet, a woman in her sixties, was under treatment for carpal tunnel syndrome, which causes numbness of the fingers. She was excited about the help she had received and was free of her symptoms. She confided that she had only one problem left in her life, and that was her husband's snoring, which disturbed her greatly. I suggested that she bring her husband in for a check-up, which she did the following week.

Ray, also in his sixties, was in surprisingly good health, and only one abnormality was found during the examination. He was allergic to wheat. Ray was given concentrated plant enzymes to be taken prior to each meal, and instructions to eliminate all wheat products from his diet for the next two weeks. Since his wife Violet did all the cooking for the family, she ensured that Ray ate no wheat. Within three days the snoring stopped.

Since one of the symptoms of allergy is a swelling of membranes, it appears that Ray must have experienced this swelling in the membranes along the roof of the mouth. As he breathed in while sleeping, the air rippled across these swollen membranes producing the loud snoring noise.

After about a month, while continuing to take his enzymes, Ray was able to include wheat in his diet again without a return of the snoring.

## Facts about Cooked Foods

Many doctors still dispute the fact that diet is related to any kind of disease. But how could diet not be involved? In order for a human cell to survive, it needs the correct pH, temperature and supply of oxygen, minerals and nutrients. Nutrients can come only from diet. If these needs of the cell are not met, changes to the cell occur. If enough cells change, tissues begin to change, then organs. Organ changes bring on functional changes with far reaching effects in the body. Knowledgeable doctors have written volumes on how nutrients are related to the common illnesses of the day, especially chronic degenerative disease such as heart disease, arthritis, diabetes, cancer and allergies. In 1982, the National Academy of Sciences estimated that 60 percent of women's cancers and 40 percent of men's cancers are related to diet. The most common cancers in this case are breast and uterine cancer, prostate cancer and gastrointestinal cancer. With all the research available, it is becoming more and more apparent that diet indeed is a major factor in disease.

Now along comes the very radical idea that cooked food may contribute to ill health. But, you say, people have been cooking food for thousands of years. That is true. And for thousands of years people have been plagued by various types of sickness. Their ill health may not be acute, as seen in infectious disease, but may take a more insidious form such as fatigue, generalized aches and pains, ulcers, gastritis, arthritis, allergies and a shortened life span. Doctors from around the world who have studied this situation have all come to the same startling conclusion: that cooked or heat-treated foods contribute to physical degeneration and disease.

Let's look at the facts. Cooking food can either destroy or make unavailable up to 85 percent of the original nutrients; it destroys 100 percent of the enzymes. Cooking protein foods can convert the proteins into new forms which are either toxic or less digestible than the raw form. This stresses the digestive organs to produce more and more enzymes. In our diets, we have few sources of raw protein that contain the enzyme protease. We toast our nuts, we cook our meat and eggs and we pasteurize our milk and dairy products. Yet, it has been shown that raw protein is more easily digested than the coagulated, cooked form.

In natural food, fat accompanies protein. Lipase is the enzyme that is normally found in fat. Once fat is cooked, the lipase is destroyed so that your body must now produce the lipase needed. Lipase is normally produced in lesser quantity than other digestive enzymes. Eating lipase-deficient fats is a potential source of stress for the digestive tract.

When lipase is deficient, fat contained in foods may be absorbed through the intestinal wall in a less digested, adulterated form. While circulating, this fat can diminish or choke off the amount of oxygen reaching the tissues and cells.

Since fat accompanies protein in foods, few raw fats are consumed. Therefore, minimal lipase enzyme is supplied from the diet. The fact that the human body has been able to adapt to some degree to denatured, cooked food is a miracle in itself. It is no accident that restorative or health-building diets have historically all been raw food diets including raw fruit and vegetable juices. These are the builders of the body because of their enzyme and nutrient content. They allow the digestive tract to "rest" and they contribute enzymes, which results in strengthening of the immune system.

Health oriented doctors from around the world realize the importance of enzyme-rich raw foods. Here are some of their conclusions. Judge for yourself.

Research done in Europe on cooked foods was reported in the book *Fats and Oils* by Udo Erasmus. "When cooked food is eaten a defense reaction occurs in the tissues of the stomach and digestive tract. This reaction is similar to the reaction we find in infections and around tumors and involves the accumulation of white blood cells, swelling and a fever-like increase of temperature of the stomach and intestinal tissues."

Dr. M. Ted Morter, Jr. describes from a chemical standpoint what cooking does to food. He explains that the chemical bonds that hold compounds (such as foods) together are not all the same. Organically bonded molecules are loosely held together and easily broken. Inorganic or ionic bonds are tightly held together and not easily broken. These bonds must be broken by enzymes during digestion in order to make use of the elements in food. Dr. Morter reports, "When you heat covalently bonded foods to more than a 130 degrees Fahrenheit, bonds that are naturally weak are made stronger. As with strong ionic bonds, heat strengthened bonds can't be broken easily, if at all. The elements are no longer as readily accessible for assimilation."

Animals in the wild eat only raw foods with loosely bonded molecules that are easy to digest and assimilate. Wild animals do not have the high incidence of chronic degenerative disease as do humans, unless they are domesticated and fed a heat-treated diet, or unless they are exposed to environmental chemicals and pollutants.

Dr. Marshal Mandell, in his book *Five Day Allergy Relief System,* states, "Substances are formed from foods during the cooking process that are totally alien to the human system and what it was designed to handle. Heating sugar creates foreign substances and caramelizes it, making tars. Browning meat creates tars all over the meat. Nothing like these tars exists in nature. And once proteins and carbohydrates and fats are heated they turn into substances that are alien to the human body."

In his book *Victory Over Diabetes* Dr. Philpott states, "Cooking food above 118°F destroys digestive enzymes. When this happens the pancreas, salivary glands, stomach and intestines must all come to the

103

rescue and furnish digestive enzymes to break down all those substances. To do this repeatedly the body must rob, so to speak, enzymes from other glands, muscles, nerves and the blood to help in its demanding process. Eventually the glands, and this includes the pancreas, develop deficiencies of enzymes, because they have been forced to work harder due to the low level of enzymes found in cooked food." Dr. Philpott supports this idea with a study done at the University of Minnesota. Rats were given an 80 percent cooked food diet for 155 days. When examined, the pancreatic weight of the rats had increased by 20 to 30 percent. There was a simultaneous decrease of digestive enzyme secretion.

The fact is that in study after study done on animals where one group is fed cooked food and the other group is fed raw food, the results are the same. The group receiving cooked food demonstrates illness and deteriorates faster. Attempts to live on the wrong kinds of fuel burden the organs and tissues beyond their capacity to maintain health.

The most famous studies ever done on the cooked food versus raw food idea were performed by Dr. Francis M. Pottenger, Jr. between 1932 and 1942 on cats. Pottenger's studies spanned ten years of cat generations and involved 900 cats. There is no similar experiment in current medical literature. Dr. Pottenger describes his findings. "Normal cats on a raw food cod-liver oil diet, show no evidence of allergy or hypothyroidism and their offspring, generation after generation, show no evidence of allergy or hypothyroidism. The incidence of these deficiency problems corresponds with the introduction of cooked foods. In giving cats cooked meat and milk they develop all kinds of allergies. They sneeze, wheeze and scratch. They are irritable, nervous and do not purr. First deficient generation allergic cats produce second generation kittens with greater incidence of allergies. And by the third generation the incidence is almost 100 percent. When second generation allergic animals are bred after being returned to an optimum raw food diet, their allergic symptoms begin to diminish and by the fourth generation, some cats show no evidence of allergy." The second and third generation of cats eating cooked meat showed abnormal respiratory tissues with edema, bronchitis and pneumonitis prevalent. Skin lesions and allergies were frequent and progressively worse from one generation to another. The intestinal tracts of several hundred normal and deficient adult cats were compared at autopsy. Measurement of the lengths of the gastrointestinal tracts were made. In a normal cat fed a raw diet, the intestinal tract was approximately 48 inches long. In the allergic cats the intestinal tracts could measure as long as 72 to 80 inches. These elongated tracts lacked tissue tone and elasticity. Based on his clinical experience and years of experiments Dr. Pottenger states, "We do know that ordinary cooking denatures proteins rendering them less easily digested. Probably certain albuminoids and globulins are physiologically destroyed. All tissue enzymes are heat labile and so destroyed. Vitamin C and some members of the B-complex are injured by the process of cooking and minerals are made less soluble by altering their physiological states."

Three indications that cooked foods are inferior are:

1. Pancreatic hypertrophy;
2. Digestive leukocytosis; and
3. Loss of enzymes and nutrients.

In judging what is an adequate diet just looking at calories, protein, carbohydrates, fats, vitamins, minerals and fiber is not enough. Availability of nutrients and enzyme content must also be considered, and the diet should be shown to sustain health generation after generation. Presence or absence of degenerative disease and length of life must also be considerations.

Food enzymes contained in raw foods can be absorbed by the human digestive tract, stored in the body and used at a later time. The fact that enzymes can be absorbed through the intestinal tract has been proven through numerous experiments. For instance, the oral use of proteolytic enzymes for sports injuries has been documented extensively. In the book *Enzyme Therapy*, Max Wolf, MD and Carl Ransberger, PhD relate an experiment using enzymes tagged with radioactive dye given to rabbits. The active enzyme molecules were later recovered in the serum, liver, kidney and urine. Enzymes are absorbed from the intestine into the lymph system and later stored in the liver and spleen. There is evidence that enzymes are circulated and secreted over and over. Therefore, they have the potential to be used more than once before being "worn out" and excreted in the urine. The important point is that by eating raw foods you help replenish the body's stores of enzymes by lowering the demand for enzymes from the digestive organs. Dr. Howell considers enzymes to be the "true yardstick of vitality." The more enzymes, the longer the life; the less enzymes, the sooner disease, old age and death result.

## CASE STUDY: *Donna*

Donna, age 37, appeared to be allergic to many things when I first saw her in my office. She stated that when she ate something to which she was allergic she would have an anaphylactic shock reaction. These reactions were preceded by dizziness, vomiting and severe abdominal pain. As a precaution, she carried epinephrine and a syringe in her purse for emergencies. Some of the foods she had previously reacted to included lettuce, cabbage, onions, peas, beans, walnuts, mustard, MSG (monosodium glutamate), shellfish, all grains, chocolate and tomatoes. Examination of this patient revealed numerous allergies, hiatus hernia and structural misalignments. In addition she was suffering from a severe Candida overgrowth infection. Donna was given a herbal liquid formula to help heal the intestinal lining, a B-complex formula with chromium, *Lactobacillus acidophilus* to help reculture the bowel, an adrenal formula, an anti-Candida formula and pancreatic enzymes. She received chiropractic adjustments once a week.

Donna was an intelligent woman eager to follow instructions. She responded well from the beginning. She had excellent follow-through on the diet and supplement program, and was prudent and knowledgeable about food choices. Her body strengthened rapidly and within two months she was able to expand her diet. After four months she had no further food reactions and was feeling great all the time. Her energy level was vastly improved. After six months of treatment she was able to eat everything without reactions, except she was afraid to try a salad. Six months later she finally "got up her nerve" to eat a salad and was delighted when "nothing happened." At this time she did not require any nutrient supplements other than

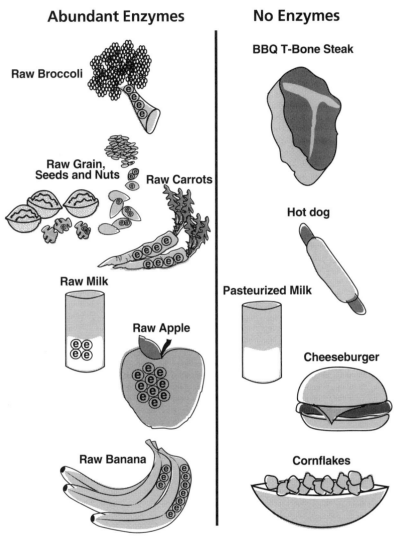

**Abundant Enzymes**

Raw Broccoli

Raw Grain, Seeds and Nuts

Raw Carrots

Raw Milk

Raw Apple

Raw Banana

**No Enzymes**

BBQ T-Bone Steak

Hot dog

Pasteurized Milk

Cheeseburger

Cornflakes

ⓔ = Enzyme

*Raw foods are enzyme-rich
cooked foods contain no enzymes*

*Figure 5.* **Enzyme Content of Foods**

concentrated plant enzymes. In the three years that I followed the case, she never had another recurrence of anaphylactic shock.

Eating more food than necessary for body functions uses up vast quantities of enzymes. This was demonstrated with an experiment done on rats. One group having unrestricted food intake, lived 483 days. The other group with partially restricted food intake lived 894 days, nearly twice as long. Consider this: 50 percent of the daily production of protein in the body is made into enzymes and a major part of this is digestive enzymes. Lowering the intake of cooked foods means less digestive enzymes are used. This helps ensure that there are sufficient metabolic enzymes at work to keep the body running efficiently and healthfully.

Only one kind of food contains enzymes: raw food. A diet of 70 percent raw food and 30 percent everything else is a vast improvement over the enzyme-deficient diet that the majority of people consume.

Vitamin $B_6$ is a precursor to at least 50 enzymes and is needed for the metabolism of all amino acids. Enzymes are built from amino acids, which makes vitamin $B_6$ a very essential part of enzyme production. Trace minerals must also be present for enzyme production. Magnesium is the mineral in greatest demand. *Clinical Ecology* states, "Maladaptive allergic and allergic-like reactions can likely be characterized by enzymatic deficiencies and when the immunological tissues are involved, antibodies are formed as a last stand at organismic survival. Nutrients are precursors to enzymes. Therefore, cellular malnutrition is the basis of these maladaptive reactions."

There are three ways to increase the enzyme content of your body.
1. Eat less food in general.
2. Eat more raw food.
3. Supplement with plant enzyme capsules. Plant enzymes ensure digestion of food and relieve the pancreas of its burden to produce 100 percent of the enzymes needed for digestion.

## Enzymes 2,000 Years Ago

*The Essene Gospel of Peace,* a compilation of third century Aramaic manuscripts and old Slavonic texts, was translated recently by

# Active Plant Enzyme pH Range

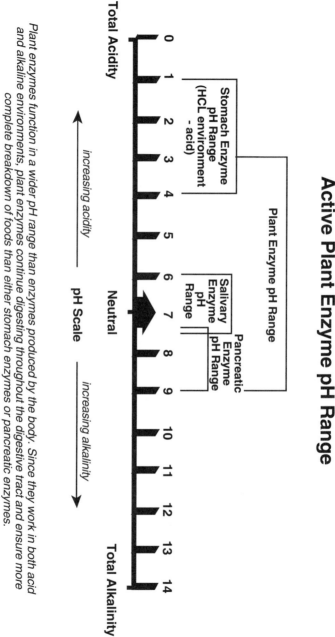

**Figure 6. Active Plant Enzyme pH Range**

Plant enzymes function in a wider pH range than enzymes produced by the body. Since they work in both acid and alkaline environments, plant enzymes continue digesting throughout the digestive tract and ensure more complete breakdown of foods than either stomach enzymes or pancreatic enzymes.

Edmond Bordeaux Szekely. In this book, Jesus counsels his followers on matters of health. Although this advice is nearly 2,000 years old, it is interesting to compare it to modern scientific knowledge of enzymes. The following are quotes from this book:

> *"So eat always from the table of God. The fruits of the trees, the grain and grasses of the field, the milk of the breasts, and the honey of the bees."* – In the natural state, all these foods are high in enzyme content.

> *"Never eat until fullness . . . so give heed to how much you have eaten when your body is sated and always eat less by a third."* – Digestive enzymes are spared by eating less.

> *"Be content with two or three sorts of food which you will always find upon the table of our earthly mother."* – Not eating too many different kinds of food at one sitting promotes digestion and spares enzymes.

> *"For if you eat living food, the same will quicken you, but if you kill your food, the dead food will kill you also, for life comes from only life, and from death comes always death. For everything which kills your foods, kills your bodies also."* – Eating raw foods with live enzymes helps produce health and longevity.

> *"Cook not, neither mix all things with one another."* – Mixing several kinds of foods in the stomach uses more enzymes.

We can recognize that the advice Jesus gave in *The Essene Gospel of Peace* is enzyme-sparing and enzyme-protecting. A high level of tissue enzymes in the body helps promote healthy tissues.

# 12

# Concern about Calcium

Experts all agree that milk is the number one allergen. Medical textbooks on pediatrics also acknowledge the allergenicity of milk to babies and children. However, the first question that a patient will ask when told they are allergic to milk is, "Where will I get my calcium?" Although logical, this question is strange from the point of view that calcium is really no more or less important than some other minerals. For example, the mineral potassium is essential for every cell in the body. A severe deficiency will cause the heart to stop beating. Yet I seldom hear the question, "Where will I get my potassium?" This over-concern about calcium has been stimulated by radio, television and magazines, primarily in commercials and advertisements for milk, cheese and antacids. These sources teach that calcium is necessary for healthy bones and for prevention of osteoporosis. While this may be true, at the same time it has been oversimplified.

Osteoporosis is certainly a legitimate concern, especially for women. One in three women will lose enough bone mineral to cause fractures. This results in over 200,000 deaths annually. However, recent studies show that boosting calcium intake may not be the answer. There are many other factors involved.

Let's first explore some of the ways that calcium may be lost from the body. If you were in a boat that had sprung a leak, wouldn't it make sense to plug the hole first? Similarly, there are many ways that calcium is drained from the body.

**Coffee, tea, soda pop and chocolate:** Intake of caffeine causes increased calcium loss in the urine.

**Refined sugar:** Ingestion of sugar increases calcium loss through urine. When foods containing calcium are taken with sugar, the absorption of usable calcium through the intestine is greatly reduced. Dr. J. B. Orr demonstrates that rickets, a calcium deficiency causing deformed bones in children, can be induced by the use of sweetened condensed milk. Many junk foods are a high source of sugar.

**Phosphorus:** Meat, grain and soft drinks have a high phosphorus content. Phosphorus binds with calcium. Therefore, when phosphorus is high in the blood, it can pull calcium from the bones. An excess intake of phosphorus results in secondary hyperparathyroidism (over-active parathyroid). A diet high in phosphorus has the same effect as a calcium deficiency. A cheeseburger with french fries and a glass of milk has 1,230 milligrams of phosphorus. The RDA of phosphorus for adults is 800 milligrams per day. On the other hand, too little phosphorus can also be detrimental. This is because calcium and phosphorus must be present in a specific ratio in order to work properly. Robert M. Giller, MD in his book *Medical Makeover* writes: "Sugar decreases the amount of phosphorus in the blood to such a degree that for two to five hours after a sugar snack, the body cannot sustain calcification."

**Salt:** Sodium, such as found in table salt increases urinary calcium excretion.

**Fiber:** A high fiber diet will decrease calcium absorption through the intestine. Many people add fiber to an already deficient diet, which can actually make their mineral absorption worse. This is due to the fact that minerals tend to bind to the fiber, becoming unavailable for use.

**Vitamin D:** Without vitamin D calcium cannot be utilized for bone formation. Vitamin D activates the absorption or transportation of calcium. Major food sources are eggs, liver and mushrooms. The sun is another source. Moderate sun exposure (approximately 20 minutes per day) is beneficial for most people.

**Protein** depletes calcium in two ways. High intake of protein causes loss of calcium through negative calcium balance. When we eat more protein than we need, the excess protein is broken down in the liver to urea. Urea has a diuretic action on the kidney which results in minerals, including calcium, being lost in the urine. Also, excess protein is acid-forming, often pulling calcium from the bones to buffer the excess acidity. Most adults take in 100 to 125 grams of protein a day. John A. McDougall, MD reports on one long-term study which measured calcium balance and found that when 75 grams of protein a day was consumed along with 1400 milligrams of calcium, "More calcium was lost in the urine than was absorbed into the body from the diet (a negative calcium balance)." High protein consumption contributes more to depletion of calcium from bones than does a deficiency of calcium intake.

Other things that contribute to a loss of calcium from the body are smoking, alcohol consumption, history of gastrointestinal surgery or malabsorption problems and taking corticosteroid medications. It is apparent that body calcium is dependent upon habits, health and lifestyle. Simply taking the RDA of 800 mg of calcium daily will not necessarily ensure that you have enough calcium. You can increase or decrease the amount of calcium your body requires by the choices you make. Before concerning yourself with taking more calcium, it may be necessary to "plug the leaky boat."

Additionally, there are several myths about calcium, particularly surrounding the consumption of milk, which must be examined.

## Calcium Myth One:
### *Milk is good for everybody.*
**Fact:** Milk is the number one allergic food. An estimated thirty-three million Americans are allergic to milk. Milk contains more than 25 different proteins that may induce allergic reaction. In addition, at least 60 million people in North America are lactose intolerant. Lactose intolerance is the inability to digest lactose, the sugar naturally present in milk. Lactase is the enzyme necessary to break down milk sugar. Most people stop manufacturing this enzyme between early childhood and adolescence. This is why 70 percent of the world pop-

ulation is lactase deficient. Perhaps this should be a tip-off that adults are not intended to drink milk. It is possible that this lack of lactase is not a deficiency, but rather the way things are naturally supposed to be. Lactose intolerance is the most common cause of gas, bloating, abdominal cramping and diarrhea.

This was an example of what can happen when only one enzyme is missing. How about a multiple enzyme deficiency? If food can't be digested, its nutrients cannot be absorbed and used.

Milk may actually create a calcium deficiency. In a lactase deficient person, the lactose ferments in the intestine because it cannot be completely broken down. When it ferments it produces lactic acid, which is absorbed into the blood stream and subsequently binds with calcium and magnesium making these minerals potentially unavailable to the tissues. Remember, calcium is the most abundant alkaline mineral used by the body to counteract acidity. Calcium is used as a buffer to protect organs from the toxic effects of caffeine, alcohol and drugs.

## Calcium Myth Two:
### Dairy products help prevent osteoporosis.
**Fact:** Milk loses 50 percent of its available calcium during pasteurization. Low fat and skim milk make calcium unavailable because fat is necessary for the proper transportation and absorption of calcium. According to a report in the *Journal of Nutrition* (February 1989), the calcium in cheese is even less available for utilization than the calcium in other dairy products. As far as osteoporosis is concerned, keep in mind that vegetarians have been shown to have higher bone density than meat eaters of the same age. Also, countries that consume the most dairy products have the most osteoporosis. Nutritionists agree that the best diet to prevent osteoporosis is a low protein, low fat, high complex carbohydrate diet that includes abundant fresh vegetables and fruit, whole grains and fresh raw seeds and nuts.

## Calcium Myth Three:
### Calcium supplementation helps prevent osteoporosis.
**Fact:** This depends on whether you have plugged the leaky boat.

Have you lowered your protein intake to the recommended level of 35 to 50 grams daily? Have you eliminated sugar, coffee, tea and soda pop from your diet? Are you eating abundant fresh fruits and vegetables? If so, calcium supplementation may not be necessary. However, if you wish to supplement, some forms of calcium are more absorbable than others. Huge doses are undesirable because less absorption takes place when too much calcium is taken at once.

Calcium is absorbed as follows: *Calcium citrate* is 50 percent calcium and probably the best absorbed calcium. *Calcium hydroxapetite* is 24 percent calcium and is also very well absorbed. *Calcium carbonate*, used in many antacids, is 50 percent calcium. *Calcium lactate*, found in milk, is best absorbed by people who are not allergic or intolerant to milk. It is 13 percent calcium. *Calcium gluconate*, which is usually well absorbed, is 9 percent calcium. *Calcium orotate* and *chelate* are approximately 10 percent calcium and are usually well-absorbed. *Bone meal* and *dolomite* have the lowest absorption and are questionable as they have frequently been shown to contain pollutants such as aluminum and lead. If you are going to take a supplement, a formula of calcium with other minerals is the safest choice so as not to deplete other minerals or upset the mineral balance. No mineral in the body works alone. Each affects the other. As we have seen, there are many factors to consider in relation to calcium.

Milk is not necessarily the answer to obtaining enough calcium. If you are allergic to milk, it definitely is not the answer. If you cannot digest milk, you cannot absorb its calcium. The milk I described here is the homogenized, pasteurized product found in supermarket dairy cases. This is a processed food with its enzymes destroyed. It requires your body to donate an enormous amount of enzymes to digest it.

Fat free milk is not without problems either. When the fat is removed the same amount of milk is higher in protein, which may cause or contribute to a negative calcium balance. Fat free milk still contains allergenic proteins and indigestible sugars.

Unpasteurized raw milk contains an enzyme which splits the calcium from the phosphorus it is bound to, making the calcium more available to the human body. Raw milk is also a high enzyme product, requiring far less of your own body's enzymes to digest it.

## Sources of Calcium

It is possible to get enough calcium in your diet without using dairy products. The following list of non-dairy foods shows that daily calcium requirements can be met without using whole cow's milk which contains only 288 mg of calcium per cup.

**Seeds and Nuts:**

| | |
|---|---|
| 1 cup sesame seeds | 2,200 mg calcium |
| 1 cup almonds | 600 mg calcium |
| 1 cup filberts (hazelnuts) | 424 mg calcium |
| 1 cup sunflower seeds | 260 mg calcium |
| 1 cup walnuts | 216 mg calcium |

**Nut Butters:**

| | |
|---|---|
| 3 oz. sesame butter | 843 mg calcium |
| 3 oz. almond butter | 225 mg calcium |
| 3 oz. filbert (hazelnut) butter | 159 mg calcium |
| 3 oz. sunflower seed butter | 99 mg calcium |
| 3 oz. cashew butter | 36 mg calcium |
| 3 oz. peanut butter | 15 mg calcium |

Note: Peanut butter is not recommended as it delivers the least calcium and is the most allergenic.

**Nut Milk** makes a good substitute for cow's milk as it is very high in calcium and a good source of essential fatty acids necessary for health. Nut milks can be used on cereals, in recipes, or for drinking from a glass. A nut milk made from two ounces of sesame seeds and two ounces of almonds will contain 712 mg of calcium per cup. Nut milk containing three ounces of sesame seed and two tablespoons of Barbados molasses will yield approximately 940 mg of calcium per cup. See recipes in Chapter 13.

Since the calcium in nut milks has not been heated or cooked, it is highly absorbable and can be easily digested. Another way to add calcium to foods is to sprinkle sesame seeds on cereals, salads, casseroles and all vegetable dishes.

## Vegetables - 1/2 cup portions:

| | |
|---|---|
| lamb's quarters | 232 mg calcium |
| collard greens | 74 mg calcium |
| turnip greens | 53 mg calcium |
| mustard greens | 52 mg calcium |
| swiss chard | 51 mg calcium |
| okra | 50 mg calcium |
| kale | 47 mg calcium |
| parsley | 39 mg calcium |
| green beans | 29 mg calcium |
| asparagus (six spears) | 22 mg calcium |
| green peas | 22 mg calcium |
| broccoli | 21 mg calcium |
| watercress | 20 mg calcium |
| cabbage | 18 mg calcium |
| spinach | 16 mg calcium |
| 1 medium artichoke | 47 mg calcium |
| 1 medium avocado | 19 mg calcium |
| 1 medium carrot | 19 mg calcium |

## Molasses:

| | |
|---|---|
| 1 tbsp. blackstrap molasses | 137 mg calcium |
| 1 tbsp. Barbados molasses | 49 mg calcium |

## Beans and Rice - 1 cup portions:

| | |
|---|---|
| soybeans | 460 mg calcium |
| tofu | 258 mg calcium |
| navy beans | 128 mg calcium |
| three bean salad | 88 mg calcium |
| pinto beans | 82 mg calcium |
| garbanzo beans (chick peas) | 80 mg calcium |
| kidney beans | 50 mg calcium |
| wild rice | 30 mg calcium |
| brown rice | 23 mg calcium |

### Seaweed - 3 ½ oz portions:

| | |
|---|---|
| wakame | 150 mg calcium |
| irish moss | 72 mg calcium |
| kelp | 68 mg calcium |
| agar | 54 mg calcium |

**Fish:** Because of the bones in canned fish, three ounces of sardines yields approximately 375 mg of calcium and three ounces of salmon yields about 203 mg of calcium.

# 13

# Fats, Oils and Allergy

Fats and oils are probably the most misunderstood and controversial of all the dietary nutrients. So much information and misinformation has become available about fats that it is difficult for interested people to sort out the facts. How fats relate to allergy has been even more of a mystery.

Why cholesterol, just one of many fatty substances, has been disproportionally singled out as the culprit in diseases involving fats is beyond comprehension. With this focus on cholesterol, the majority of people are unaware of the effects of toxic *trans-* fatty acids and harmful free radicals which have a proven record of damage to human tissues.

Since 75 percent of the North American population dies prematurely of diseases related to fats, learning which fats to use, which to avoid and what fats do in the body becomes an absolute prerequisite to maintaining good health. In addition, today's fats and oils have a surprising connection to allergy. Fats are the only food group not absorbed into the blood from the intestinal lining. Instead, they are broken down into fatty acids and absorbed into the lymphatics. Here they are circulated and eventually enter the blood stream. Fats alone seldom trigger allergic reactions. Although milk is a highly allergenic food, butter seldom causes an allergic reaction. However, many commonly eaten fats pave the way for inflammatory or allergic reactions.

This is why it is so important to identify these fats and eliminate them from the diets of people with allergies. There is no point in feeding an inflammatory reaction in the body of an individual whose body is already compromised with allergies.

There are only two fatty acids that are considered essential to life. They are essential because they cannot be manufactured in the body and must be obtained from the diet. These two fatty acids are called linoleic (LA or Omega 6) and linolenic (LNA or Omega 3). Sources of LA include safflower, sunflower, corn, soy and sesame oils. The best source of LNA is flaxseed oil. Both of these fatty acids play important roles in protecting your cardiovascular system and heart from atherosclerosis.

That is only one reason why these fatty acids are important. They are also converted into hormone-like substances in your body called prostaglandins. Prostaglandins act as messengers and regulate vital metabolic processes throughout the body. About 30 prostaglandins have been discovered to date. There are three major categories or families of prostaglandins. Prostaglandins act like a check and balance system in the body. For every action of one prostaglandin there is a prostaglandin that performs the opposite action. For example, if one prostaglandin were to turn on the water faucet, there would be another prostaglandin to turn it off. Keeping them in balance is important. Consider our "water faucet" prostaglandins: one prostaglandin turns on the water, but the other prostaglandin is disabled and cannot turn it off. The water overflows the sink. What if another prostaglandin comes along and turns on another faucet and the disabled prostaglandin still cannot turn it off? The whole house could be flooded. Similar events happen in your body when you eat the wrong kinds of fat. To allergy sufferers the prostaglandins that play a role in controlling inflammation are the most important. For instance, LNA (Omega 3) helps control allergic manifestation in the skin in the form of eczema.

Inflammation in the body is not always bad. It is a normal and natural part of the healing process. When you have a cut in the skin, it is the inflammatory process that calls the appropriate cells to the area to heal the wound. Inflammation out of control is destructive.

Prostaglandins can either create inflammation or inhibit it. Inflammation running wild is part of allergic reactions. It can be controlled depending on what type of fat is fed to the body.

There are basically two kinds of fats, saturated and unsaturated. Saturated fat is solid at room temperature and comes mainly from animal sources. Unsaturated fat is liquid at room temperature and comes from vegetable sources. The fatty acid LA converts to the prostaglandin 1 family (called PG1) whose effects are preventing inflammation, blocking allergic responses and enhancing the immune system. The fatty acid LNA converts to the prostaglandin 3 family (PG3) which also prevents inflammation and enhances the immune system. PG3 blocks the release of inflammatory products from the mast cells and basophils that are involved in allergic reactions.

The prostaglandin 2 family (PG2) has the opposite effect. It promotes inflammation, suppresses the immune system and stimulates the allergic response. PG2 is built from a fatty acid known as arachidonic acid. Sources of arachidonic acid are meat, milk and eggs. You can see at once that most people eat far more meat, milk and eggs than they do flaxseed oil. That is why in some allergic individuals it is necessary to limit or eliminate those foods in order to bring inflammation under control. In other words, removal of these foods from the diet stops feeding the inflammatory pathway. (See Figure 7, page 122.)

Addition of flaxseed oil to the diet feeds the anti-allergic, anti-inflammatory pathway. Did you ever notice a big flare-up of symptoms one to three days after eating a big steak dinner or a pizza (meat and milk products)? Or perhaps you are eating meat, milk and eggs on a daily basis and have continual or chronic inflammation. These arachidonic acid foods load up your cells with inflammatory substances. When the allergic reaction takes place, the cell membrane breaks releasing these inflammatory substances and causing tissue damage. It makes sense for people who are prone to allergy to restrict foods that feed inflammatory reactions. Leukotrienes are one substance made from arachidonic acid. They are 1,000 to 10,000 times more inflammatory than histamine. Leukotrienes are often involved in allergic reactions.

# Important Pathways

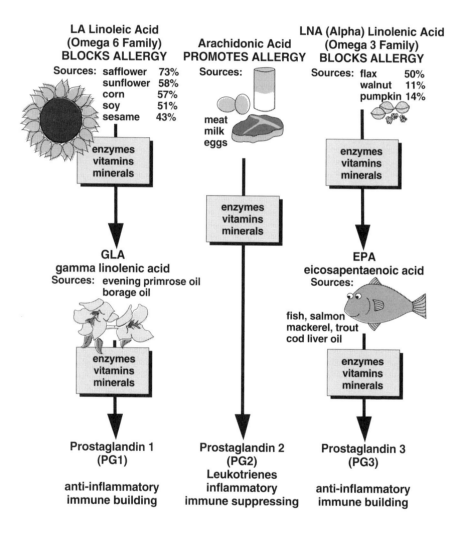

| LA Linoleic Acid (Omega 6 Family) BLOCKS ALLERGY | Arachidonic Acid PROMOTES ALLERGY | LNA (Alpha) Linolenic Acid (Omega 3 Family) BLOCKS ALLERGY |

Sources: safflower 73% / sunflower 58% / corn 57% / soy 51% / sesame 43%

Sources: meat milk eggs

Sources: flax 50% / walnut 11% / pumpkin 14%

enzymes vitamins minerals

enzymes vitamins minerals

enzymes vitamins minerals

**GLA** gamma linolenic acid
Sources: evening primrose oil borage oil

**EPA** eicosapentaenoic acid
Sources: fish, salmon mackerel, trout cod liver oil

enzymes vitamins minerals

enzymes vitamins minerals

enzymes vitamins minerals

**Prostaglandin 1 (PG1)**
anti-inflammatory immune building

**Prostaglandin 2 (PG2) Leukotrienes**
inflammatory immune suppressing

**Prostaglandin 3 (PG3)**
anti-inflammatory immune building

*Figure 7.* Important Pathways

It sounds simple. Cut back or eliminate foods that encourage inflammation and add the inflammation-fighting oils into your diet. But there is more. Fats are converted to fatty acids and prostaglandins by a series of steps that involves enzymes, vitamins and minerals. If any of these factors are missing, the conversion cannot take place. One necessary and important enzyme is called Delta 6 desaturase. It can be inactivated by several common factors, including drugs such as cortisone, alcohol, tobacco, excess saturated fat in the diet and heated fats such as the fats in fried food. When these factors are present, Delta 6 desaturase cannot convert beneficial oils into anti-inflammatory prostaglandins. Although inflammation is a normal and necessary part of the healing reaction, wild, unchecked inflammation is destructive and tissue-damaging. This is attested to by the millions of dollars spent every year on anti-inflammatory drugs.

What people do not understand is that the body produces its own anti-inflammatory substances in the form of prostaglandins. All it needs is the necessary raw materials from foods with which to work.

In order to make good choices, it is essential to learn about the proper oils and how to obtain them. You are probably familiar with the fact that white sugar is a refined product. Refined sugar is stripped of its nutrients with only the carbohydrates left. White flour is also a nutrient-poor, refined product. Unfortunately, it is no different for oils. The safflower oil sitting on the supermarket shelf has been refined and the LA it contained has been virtually destroyed in the manufacturing process.

When oil is refined several toxic products are formed. Among them are *trans-* fatty acids. Fats and oils are very sensitive to light, heat and oxygen. You cannot heat or cook any kind of oil without producing toxic by-products. Commercial oils of safflower, corn and sunflower have been heated to temperatures of 464 to 518°F for 30 to 60 minutes, forming *trans-* fatty acids. The very molecules of the oil have been denatured. They have been forced into a new, unnatural shape, becoming straight, while the normal shape is curved or horseshoe-shaped. The problem is that these abnormal, straightened molecules do not fit into the biological membranes of the cells in the same way as the horseshoe-shaped molecules. It is like trying to put the wrong piece in a jigsaw puzzle: it just doesn't fit. The molecules of the refined oil only partially fit the cell membranes. They take up the space, but can't do the work. The worst damaging effect is that *trans-* fatty acids block out natural healthful fat so that it cannot function. *Trans-* fatty acids get incorporated into many tissues, including the heart, whose normal fuel is fatty acids. Since enzymes break down the *trans-* fatty acids more slowly than the natural horseshoe-shaped fatty acids, impaired function may result.

Another destructive aspect of *trans-* fatty acids is that, while residing in unsaturated fat, they act more like saturated fat. *Trans-* fatty acids are sticky and cause blood cells to clump together. They can cause fatty deposits in blood vessels by altering cholesterol metabolism. *Trans-* fatty acids are powerful immune-system inhibitors that block enzymes which help the production of prostaglandins. Since they displace natural fats at the cell membrane, they reduce oxygen supply to the cell. On the other hand, natural fats attract oxygen, which is their normal physiological function.

The nervous system consists primarily of fat tissue. *Trans-* fatty acids help promote degeneration of nerves. *Trans-* fatty acids can trigger the release of inflammatory arachidonic acid products from cells. Worst of all, *trans-* fatty acids disrupt the vital activities of the natural fats and create a deficiency of the fatty acids essential for life: LA and LNA.

There is even more bad news. *Trans-* fatty acids are found in nearly all packaged and processed foods. If the package says "hydrogenated" or "partially-hydrogenated" vegetable oil, it contains *trans-* fatty acids. The average intake of *trans-* fatty acids is about twelve grams per day, which is nearly twice as much as all the other food additives put together.

Major sources of *trans-* fatty acids are margarine, vegetable oil and shortening. Stick margarine averages 31 percent *trans-* fatty acids, but can be as high as 47 percent. Vegetable oil shortenings may contain over 37 percent *trans-* fatty acids. In contrast, European oils cannot contain more than 1 percent *trans-* fatty acids, and the Dutch government has banned the sale of margarine containing *trans-* fatty acids.

Margarine is simply not the healthful product that the public has been led to believe it is. In addition to *trans-* fatty acids, it contains dozens of other toxic compounds produced by the hydrogenation process and by the heat, light and oxygen that its oils are exposed to in the refining process. Recent studies show that margarine may actually raise blood cholesterol levels.

The amounts of essential fatty acids that margarine contains have been greatly reduced by the refining process. Udo Erasmus, author of *Fats and Oils* states "Margarines, the way they are now manufactured, are dangerous to health, especially when consumed to excess."

Studies show that it takes over seven weeks to remove half of the *trans-* fatty acids from the heart. *Trans-* fatty acids can be removed by increasing consumption of LNA, found in flaxseed oil, while simultaneously decreasing intake of products containing *trans-* fatty acids.

Other common products that contain *trans-* fatty acids are:

| Product | % *Trans-* Fatty Acids |
| --- | --- |
| salad oil | 13% |
| french fries | 37% |
| candies, cookies, frostings | 30-40% |
| bread and rolls | (up to) 24% |
| doughnuts and pastries | (up to) 33% |
| crackers | 20-30% |
| corn chips | 24-34% |

In addition to the oils already mentioned, two beneficial oils that can be used to supplement the diet are evening primrose oil and fish oil. Evening primrose oil contains gamma-linoleic acid (GLA). It is normally formed from LA. It follows the anti-inflammatory PG1 pathway. Fish oil is the main source of eicosapentaenoic acid (EPA). EPA is normally formed from LNA. EPA displaces arachidonic acid, keeping blood free-flowing. It also has anti-inflammatory properties. Cold water fish such as mackerel contain EPA. Scallops contain 20 percent EPA. Oysters and red caviar are also good sources. EPA is found in cod-liver oil.

An important point to remember is that LA and LNA are natural fats designed to do life-supporting work in the body. *Trans-* fatty acids are the by-products in man-made processed foods. *Trans-* fatty acids are foreign to, and cannot be beneficially used by, the body.

Another major problem with fats that have been heated to high temperatures, either in the refining process or by frying, is the formation of free radicals. Simply speaking, free radicals are highly reactive molecules which move with lightning speed through the body. They are a primary cause of cellular damage, "old age skin spots" and wrinkling of the skin. Free radicals damage the outer membranes of the cells so that they cannot hold tightly together, causing the skin to sag or wrinkle. In severe damage, the cells die and rise to the skin surface, forming the brown skin spots we see in elderly people. High fat diets and chemical toxins encourage the process of cellular damage by free radicals. These highly reactive molecules can also be formed by exposing the body to external sources of radiation.

Cells can be protected from free radical damage by avoiding both internal and external causes of free radical formation. Common sources of free radicals include refined and rancid fats, fried food, chemical pollutants and radiation.

Essential fatty acid deficiency is probably the most common, but least recognized, nutritional deficiency. This deficiency leads to immune system breakdown setting the stage for allergy. People experiencing fatty acid deficiency are prone to allergies, sinus problems, hay fever, asthma, psoriasis, eczema, premenstrual syndrome and other conditions. Symptoms of deficiency include:

| | |
|---|---|
| bleeding gums | dry, flaky skin |
| dry, brittle or oily hair | brittle nails |
| cold hands and feet | excess ear wax |
| lowered resistance to infection | hair loss |

The immune system cannot function well without essential fatty acids. In fact, it has been shown that cells and organs will degenerate if essential fatty acids are not supplied by the diet. Children are especially dependent upon LA and LNA for brain development. Besides being caused by direct deficiency in the diet, essential fatty acid deficiency can be created by common dietary practices such as:

1. Chronic intake of alcohol.
2. High intake of refined sugar.

3. Excess intake of saturated fat.
4. Intake of hydrogenated, partially hydrogenated or deep-fried fats.
5. Smoking.
6. Use of drugs such as cortisone, or the overuse of antibiotics.

Natural foods containing essential fatty acids include:

| | |
|---|---|
| nuts (raw, unsalted) | avocado |
| seeds (raw, unsalted), | cold water fish |
| especially pumpkin, | beans |
| sunflower, sesame and flax | green leafy vegetables |

Canola oil is the most unsaturated oil available on the market, and for this reason has been recently promoted as being healthful. Used in its unrefined form, this may be true. However, most canola available to the public is refined and therefore subject to forming the same toxic substances as other oils namely, *trans-* fatty acids and free radicals.

Another concern with canola has been its content of erucic acid. Through laboratory studies done with canola, erucic acid was thought to cause fatty degeneration of the heart, kidney, adrenals and thyroid of rats. Based on this assumption, new varieties of low erucic acid rapeseed were bred and government standards limited the erucic acid content of canola to 5 percent or less.

According to Udo Erasmus, author of *Fats That Heal, Fats That Kill,* it now appears that other oils such as sunflower that contains no erucic acid will cause the same degenerative changes in rats as canola. Evidently, rats do not metabolize fats and oils well and there are indications that rat metabolism in this respect may differ substantially from human fat metabolism. More recent findings indicate that canola oil will not cause the same problems in human hearts as in rat hearts. Consequently, it appears that the erucic acid content of canola is not so toxic as once believed.

Cottonseed oil is often used in margarine and mayonnaise. However, since cotton is not a food crop, chemicals banned for use on food crops are not banned for cotton. Highly toxic chemicals such as paraquat and arsenic have been used on cotton crops. Cottonseed oil may contain residues of these toxic chemicals and therefore cannot be recommended. Cottonseed oil contains cyclopropene fatty acid, which has known toxic effects on the liver and gall bladder. In addition to margarine and mayonnaise, cottonseed oil often appears in products such as crackers, salad dressing, potato chips and other chips and baking mixes.

## Using Healthful Oils

While the various metabolic pathways of fats and oils may seem complicated to the person unfamiliar with biochemistry, making use of the information about oils is fairly simple. There are only a few key points that a person must know in order to get the good elements from fats and oils and eliminate the harmful ones.

First, eliminate all fried foods. The high heat of frying alters the oil, producing *trans-* fatty acids, free radicals and other toxic products.

Second, use only unrefined oil found in dark bottles in the refrigerated portion of the health food store. Make your own salad dressings and mayonnaise with these oils. Include flax oil in the diet. If you purchase a product that already has oil added to it, you can almost be sure the oil is refined and nutrient deficient.

Third, if you sauté vegetables such as in stir-frying, use only a small quantity, one tablespoon or less, of butter or extra virgin olive oil. These are the only two fats that should ever be heated as they are more stable and produce the least toxic substances. Adding chopped onions or garlic to the fat in the pan helps protect the fat from oxidation and produces even less toxic elements. Better yet, sauté vegetables and meats in broth or pure water.

Fourth, use butter rather than margarine. Since butter is a saturated fat, it should be used in small quantities. However, it is more digestible than margarine and contains less chemicals and toxic products.

Fifth, add ground up flax seed to cereals and salads. A coffee grinder will grind a small amount for immediate use. Never store the ground-up flax seed and never cook with flaxseed oil as it becomes toxic when heated.

Sixth, get a book that tells you how much fat, in grams, you are eating each day. Keep track of this for one week. The amount of fat should not exceed 20 percent of the calories eaten. That would be 40 grams on a 2,000 calorie diet. Systematically cut fat down to this level, eliminating the sources of refined oils and adding in unrefined oils.

Good sources of LA include the unrefined oils of:

| | |
|---|---|
| safflower | 73% linoleic |
| sunflower | 58% linoleic |
| corn | 57% linoleic |
| soy | 51% linoleic |

Good sources of LNA are less common. The unrefined oil of flax seed contains 50 percent LNA. Flaxseed oil contains some LA as well, making flax oil the most important oil you can add to your diet. Other sources of LNA include:

| | |
|---|---|
| walnut oil | 11% linolenic |
| poppy seed oil | 30% linolenic |
| soybean oil | 7% linolenic |
| pumpkin seed oil | 15% linolenic |

## Tasty Ways to Use Oils

Whenever we start to use new products in new ways, there can be stumbling blocks. It takes time, effort and thought to incorporate new ideas in the kitchen. A few key recipes are included here in order to help you get started using the essential oils that are beneficial, and to show you how easy it can be to use seeds and nuts. All the recipes are easy, quick to prepare and very tasty.

### Instant Breakfast

All seeds used are raw, unsalted.
Mix together and soak in 3/4 cup of pure water for 24 hours:
1 tbsp. pumpkin seeds
1 tbsp. sesame seeds
1 tbsp. flax seed
2 tbsp. almonds
1 tbsp. sunflower seeds

Pour into blender and liquefy while adding 1 cup of water. Add two to three tsp. raw, unpasteurized honey. Add 1 to 1½ cups of frozen or fresh berries, cherries, or banana. Makes two large glasses.

129

This recipe contains the essential oils that the body can quickly burn for energy, that are necessary for brain growth and function and that help normalize cholesterol. It is also high in organic trace minerals and calcium. Ounce for ounce, sesame seeds contain more calcium than milk.

### Whole Grain Cereal

Use any organic whole grain such as millet, barley, wheat or oats. Soak 1 cup of grain in 2 cups of water for 12 hours.

When you are ready for bed, pour the grain into a casserole dish or crock pot. Bake in the oven or cook in a crock pot at the lowest setting (120 to 150°F). When you get up in the morning, the cereal is hot and ready to eat.

This cereal is chewy and tasty as is, but a variation can be made by creaming it in the blender. This will have a texture that is more familiar to children. To cream cereal, put about ½ cup cooked grain in the blender and add hot water slowly while blending until the desired consistency is reached. Cereal can be topped with raw, unpasteurized honey, molasses, cinnamon, chopped dried fruits, raisins, dates, warm apple juice, pure maple syrup or seed and nut milk. Whole grain cereal made in the above manner contains fiber, B vitamins, minerals and a small amount of essential fatty acids.

### Seed and Nut Milk Basic Recipe

½ cup raw almonds
¼ cup sesame seeds

Soak in 2 cups of pure water for 24 hours. Pour into blender and blend as you add enough water to fill the blender. Add unpasteurized honey to taste, (approximately 1 tablespoon) Add 1 teaspoon vanilla, or to taste. Pour through strainer.

Nut milk will keep in the refrigerator approximately three days. Store in a dark bottle if possible. This nut milk is high in calcium, and contains essential oils and trace minerals in a form easily utilized by the body. Any raw nuts can be used to make nut milk. However, sesame seeds and almonds are highest in calcium. Flax seed can also be added to this recipe in order to raise the content of LNA. Nut milk may be used over cereal, over berries or in recipes, or it may be drunk from a glass.

## Mayonnaise

Commercial mayonnaise is often made from cottonseed oil or other vegetable oils that have been refined at high temperatures and exposed to light and oxygen, creating many toxic by-products including *trans-* fatty acids. Through such treatment, the essential fatty acids, LA and LNA, have been degraded.

Many health authorities simply advise against eating mayonnaise at all. However, it is easy to make mayonnaise that is a healthful product which contributes essential nutrients to your diet, whether you make a sandwich to take to school or a dip to eat with vegetables. You must remember, however, that even good quality mayonnaise is nearly 100% fat and should be used in small quantities.

### Mayonnaise Recipe

1 fresh egg
5 tsp. fresh lemon juice
2 tsp. Dijon mustard
½ tsp. sea salt (optional)
Dash of Tabasco sauce

Add above ingredients to blender and blend for 5 seconds until mixed. Add one cup unrefined oil slowly in a thin stream. This oil must be labeled unrefined or cold-pressed. It should be found in a dark bottle in the refrigerator of the health food store. Safflower, sunflower or walnut oils are good oils for this recipe. Use ¾ cup safflower, sunflower or walnut oil and ¼ cup flax seed oil to include all the essential fatty acids. This mixture tastes like regular mayonnaise, but will be slightly cream colored. If the color is objectionable, eliminate the flax oil and use 1 cup of the safflower only. Store mayonnaise in the refrigerator for up to two weeks.

### Whipped Butter

Use 1 part butter to 1 part flaxseed oil. Blend softened butter and oil in blender. Store in the refrigerator up to three days. This recipe helps cut down the amount of saturated fat of the butter while adding in the essential oils necessary for health. This butter must not be used for cooking.

### Salad Dressing – Basic Recipe
¼ cup unrefined oil (combinations of safflower, sunflower, walnut and flaxseed oils are all good choices)
2 cloves fresh garlic, minced
¼ cup fresh lemon juice
Pinch of sea salt if desired
Any other seasoning you wish to add such as fresh herbs, onion, etc. or a packet of salad seasonings obtained from your health food store.
Blend together in blender. Store in refrigerator

### Avocado Dressing
1 medium avocado, ripe
2 cloves garlic, minced
2 rounded tbsp. chopped onions
¼ cup of unrefined oil
sea salt to taste
Blend in blender until smooth. Serve on salad immediately.

### Easy Caesar Dressing
½ cup unrefined oil (a mixture of safflower oil, or walnut oil, and flaxseed oil is good)
1 fresh farm egg
1 tbsp. Worcestershire sauce
⅓ cup fresh lemon juice
2 cloves garlic, coarsely chopped
pinch of sea salt
¼ tsp. freshly ground pepper
½ cup fresh grated Parmesan cheese
Optional ingredient: can of anchovies
Blend all ingredients until smooth. This recipe can be made ahead and stored in a covered, dark container in the refrigerator. It is best when made a day ahead of use.

**Vegetable Dip – Children Can Become Vegetable Lovers**
Children like small chunks of raw vegetables that they can dip. Serve vegetables to children an hour before dinner. While they are dipping, you can prepare the rest of the meal in peace. Cut up raw vegetables. Experiment with new vegetables and new shapes such as carrot curls, carved animals from turnips, cucumbers and fresh broccoli.

Use avocado dressing for dip, or make a dip using the mayonnaise recipe. Take equal quantities of mayonnaise and low- or non-fat yogurt as a base. Mix in seasonings, such as curry, onion, garlic or whatever your children enjoy.

**Vegetable Juice**
Another pre-dinner idea is to juice the vegetables. With a juicer, use carrots for a base. Good proportions are 80 percent carrot juice and 20 percent green vegetables such as celery, parsley, watercress, broccoli, cabbage, etc. If juice seems bitter, add one apple and serve. Most children will enjoy this juice if served fresh and if greens are held to a minimum at first. Then add in greater quantities of greens as they get used to the idea of drinking the vegetables. Many juice books are available at health food stores for extra ideas.

# 14

## Children and Allergies

Other than asthma, the four most common symptoms of allergy seen in children are colic in infants, ear infection, bed-wetting and hyperactivity.

### Colic

Colic is so common that newborn babies are almost expected to have it. However, James C. Breneman, MD considers it to be "a definite manifestation of intolerance, much of which is allergic." In this condition, and especially in infants whose entire diet is milk, cow's milk is overwhelmingly the leading allergen. Babies who are breast-fed may still develop allergy to cow's milk if the mother ingests milk, cheese, yogurt or other dairy products. Cow's milk proteins in the form of immune complexes can be transmitted to a baby through breast milk, causing sensitization in the infant. Intestinal biopsies have been performed on infants with colic after they were fed cow's milk for seven days. Increased IgE levels, indicating allergy, have been found in the cells of the biopsy samples.

Breast milk is in the raw state. It has not been cooked or heated, so it is a very enzyme-dense product. The enzymes contained in breast milk help the baby digest the milk, taking stress off its immature digestive tract. Infant formulas contain no enzymes and force the infant's digestive organs to do all the work. Cow's milk formula is higher in protein and fat than breast milk, giving the baby's digestive tract even more of a workout. If the baby's digestive tract is unable to produce sufficient enzymes to digest the cow's milk formula, colic will result. Since the baby's immature digestive tract is naturally more permeable than an older child's, it allows easier absorption of partially digested protein particles, leading to allergy.

Colic is easily remedied in a baby. In the breast-fed baby, the mother should eliminate all sources of dairy products from her diet. The baby should be given concentrated plant enzymes each time it is fed. For the formula-fed infant, the formulas should be rotated every four to five days from soy formula, to goat's milk formula and the various other formulas that can be found. Each time the baby is fed, concentrated plant enzymes should be supplemented.

Colic is only one symptom of food allergy in a baby. Other common symptoms include:

| | | |
|---|---|---|
| rashes | cold sores | bronchitis |
| loose bowels | fussy eater | eczema |
| frequent "colds" | hives or welts | wheezing |
| irritability | nose rubbing | bloodshot eyes |
| chronic cough | tiny broken blood | nasal stuffiness, |
| diaper rash, redness | vessels under the | sniffling, snorting, |
| at anus or on cheeks | skin | sneezing |

It is ironic that we feed the most allergenic food known to man to our babies and children. B-lactoglobulin, a substance found in cow's milk, but not in human milk, is foreign to the baby's digestive tract. Newborn babies have increased gastrointestinal permeability to B-lactoglobulin, probably because of a lack of enzymes to digest it. Casein is another of the most allergenic proteins in milk.

Allergy to milk creates gastrointestinal bleeding, leading to iron-deficiency anemia in infants due to a loss of blood in the stool. If the blood comes from high up in the intestinal tract, it will appear as dark or black and is not readily recognized. This blood loss can go undetected for long periods resulting in iron deficiency in the child. Other diseases that have been associated with milk include celiac disease, chronic diarrhea, various gastroenteropathies, pulmonary manifestations and fibrosis.

136

CASE STUDY: *Amy*

Amy was only ten months old when her mother brought her to my office. She was showing obvious signs of food allergy and had eczema. Her mother was breast feeding her as Amy could not tolerate other forms of food. She was not even doing well on the breast milk. She had frequent colic and a rash on her arms and legs. Examination of the infant showed that she was intolerant to all milk, including breast milk. She reacted strongly to tobacco smoke and sugar. There was under-functioning of the pancreas, liver and kidneys.

Treatment consisted of chiropractic adjustments to help align and balance the body. Amy was to have concentrated plant enzymes each time she ate, and a nutritional supplement daily. The mother was told to refrain from all dairy products as allergenic particles from milk can be present in the breast milk. She was told to continue breast feeding and not to introduce new foods for the time being.

Over the next few weeks, the eczema and stomach distress disappeared. After eight weeks, the mother was successfully able to introduce some fruits and vegetables into the diet. Amy continued to improve, and eight months after beginning treatment she was able to tolerate all food groups without a return of symptoms. Her pancreas, liver and kidneys tested normal. One and a half years later, Amy had had no recurrence of symptoms and was a healthy, normal youngster.

## Ear Infection – A New Epidemic

Each year ten million children in the United States are treated for middle ear infections. It has become the most common reason for surgery in children. To demonstrate the magnitude of the problem, 70 percent of all children suffer from ear infection at least once. More than half of these children suffer ear infection before their third birthday. Middle ear infection is the leading cause of deafness in children. Antibiotics are the standard treatment. However, antibiotics provide only temporary, symptomatic relief and no protection against recurring episodes.

A recent study done on the effectiveness of antibiotics for middle ear infection demonstrated that after treatment with amoxicillin 69 percent of the children still had otitis media (middle ear inflammation). Another study showed that amoxicillin administration conferred no more protection against acute episodes than a placebo.

Commonly, the child is subjected to repeated doses of antibiotics until the recommendation for tympanostomy (tubes in the ears) is finally made. While this procedure is generally regarded to be safe, it usually involves a general anesthetic, which in itself carries some risk. The tubes stay in place from three to eighteen months, with six months being average, before they are extruded into the ear canal. In some cases, the surgical procedure must be repeated two or three times. Scarring of the tympanic membrane (ear drum) and loss of hearing are side effects of tympanostomy. At best, tympanostomy is a symptomatic treatment.

Isn't there a better way? What causes ears to become inflamed over and over, and why are antibiotics and surgery not a permanent cure? Many causes have been traditionally recognized, such as blocked eustachian tube – the tiny tube that runs from the middle ear to the nasopharynx. Studies show that when this tube is blocked, the middle ear will accumulate fluid. When infections originate in the throat, nasal areas or tonsils, the pathogenic bacteria often migrate up the eustachian tube to the middle ear. In an infant or younger child the eustachian tube is short, straight and horizontal, whereas that of the adult is more angular and closed, except during the act of swallowing or yawning. This factor allows for easier infection in the infant.

Clinical studies show allergy plays a major role in middle ear infection. In a recent study of 448 patients with middle ear infection, 57 percent had asthma, a known allergic problem, 95 percent had allergic rhinitis and 16 percent had atopic dermatitis (rash). Another study showed that half of the children with allergic disease have middle ear dysfunction. A further study concluded that there is immune deficiency in children with otitis media. IgE and IgG antibodies against specific foods have been isolated in the serum and middle ear fluids of otitis-prone children. Of these antibodies, the one for milk is the most common, followed by egg, then wheat.

New studies suggest that breast feeding of infants has a protective effect against infections of the middle ear. In 256 infants, the incidence of otitis media was inversely associated with the duration of breast feeding. In other words, the longer the infant was breast fed, the less middle ear infections. A Boston study of 692 children also indicated that "Breast feeding was associated significantly with decreased risk of recurrent acute otitis media."

Why would breast feeding make such a difference? There are several explanations:

1. Allergy to one or more components in cow's or formula milk. It is well known that swelling of tissues is an effect of allergy. In this case the mucosa of the eustachian tube swells, closing the opening from the nasopharynx to the middle ear. Once the eustachian tube is blocked, fluid begins to collect in the middle ear, often resulting in infection.

2. Breast milk conveys immunological factors to the infant which help prevent bacterial and viral infections. It contains immuno globulins and various types of white blood cells. Breast milk prevents the attachment of Pneumococci and Haemophilus influenza (pneumonia- and flu-causing bacteria) to epithelial cells.

3. Breast milk is in the raw, uncooked state, which means that it contains natural enzymes to aid in its digestion, requiring little digestive effort on the part of the infant. Cow's milk and infant formulas have been heat-treated through pasteurization at temperatures high enough to kill all the enzymes. In order to digest this milk, the infant must supply all of the enzymes from its own digestive fluids. If its immature digestive tract cannot supply all the needed enzymes, incomplete digestion takes place. Partially digested protein particles can now pass through the intestinal lining and into the general circulation, causing an allergic response. The fact that IgE and IgG antibodies have been isolated in inner ear fluids indicates the ear is a site for the allergic reaction. Cow's milk and infant formulas are much higher in protein content than breast milk, putting an additional load on the infant's digestive tract and allowing more potential for incompletely digested protein to enter the general circulation.

4. Antibiotics used to treat middle ear infection can create candidiasis. Clinical studies show that Candida is usually present in the middle ear after one or two episodes of middle ear infection. A baby can also be born with this condition if the mother has candidiasis. This chronic infection keeps the ear in a weakened condition of lowered immunity and allows new infections of bacteria to occur.

## How to Help Your Child Recover from Ear Infection and Avoid Ear Tubes

Clinical studies show that nutritional therapy helps prevent recurring episodes of middle ear infection. If your child has ear infection there are specific things you can do to help. Keep in mind, however, that there are many individual differences and needs. Only the most commonly seen conditions are addressed here. If your child has had two bouts of ear infection in the first two years of life, all of the following can be helpful:

1. Supply *Lactobacillus acidophilus* to the child. Good quality products are kept in the refrigerated portion of the health food store. They come in powder or capsule form. For very young children, the powder form is best. Administer daily for a minimum of one month in mild cases of ear infection, and up to six months to one year for severe cases.

2. Give concentrated plant enzymes each time the child eats. Protease should be the first ingredient listed on the label, along with amylase, lipase and cellulase. Capsules can be opened and the contents mixed with food if the child is too young to swallow capsules.

3. Eliminate dairy products. This includes all dairy products such as milk, cheese, yogurt, ice cream, etc. Also eliminate all products containing refined sugar, peanuts and peanut butter. This alone will help the digestive tract improve function because it eliminates the foods that place the greatest demand upon it. If the child has had severe and/or frequent ear infections, assume that any frequently eaten food, such as wheat, corn or eggs can be involved allergically. These foods need only be removed for

one month. The milk and sugar products must be restricted for several months and allowed only infrequently after that period of time. Homogenized, pasteurized milk should never be allowed.

4. Use mullein oil ear drops, available at health food stores, nightly for one week. Then use the ear drops only if symptoms of ear infection should reappear. A good formula contains mullein oil, hypericum oil and garlic oil.

This program covers only the usual or common case. If your child still demonstrates symptoms after six weeks of adherence to this program, additional advice should be sought. Nearly all children with ear infection will show improvement on this program, but some children have special idiosyncrasies that must be addressed. This program has been successful with hundreds of children with no negative side effects.

## Bed-Wetting

Bed-wetting is a common problem of childhood. Recent statistics show 20 to 25 percent of children are still affected by bed-wetting at the age of six. This results in tension and anxiety for both the child and the family. The child's self-esteem often suffers. Yet medical reports indicate that there is seldom any physical abnormality with the child. The vast majority of these children have normal urinalysis and normal physical findings, including normal bladder size.

The frequency of bed-wetting tends to decrease as the child grows older with only one or two percent of cases persisting into adulthood. Medical treatment stresses control of the problem rather than treatment. Dr. Robert Schwarz, Associate Professor of Urology, associated with the Department of Pediatrics at Dalhousie University in Halifax, Nova Scotia, states, "It is not known why some children are bed-wetters." He adds that "laziness" or deliberate bed-wetting is rare and seen only in conjunction with other overt behavioral problems.

There appears to be no correlation between EEG sleep patterns and wetting episodes. Medical management centers around the use of tricyclic anti-depressants such as Imipramine. This drug apparently has some effectiveness, but parents should be aware of the side effects such as life-threatening heart rhythm disturbances in doses over 20 milligrams per kilogram of body weight. Another control method is the electric alarm system which apparently has a 75 to 90 percent success rate, but can take weeks or months to achieve a non-wetting state, depending on the child's age and ability to respond to the training measure of a buzzer. However, neither of these methods helps correct biochemical or allergic problems which may be present.

The usual case history is that of an apparently healthy child with no diagnosed physical disturbances of the bladder or urethra, no current urinary infections and no known neurological symptoms. There is often a family history of bed-wetting, on one or both parents' sides. The child toilet trains at a normal age and has no daytime wetting problems. Frequency of bed-wetting ranges from nightly or several times per week to several times per month.

Clinical experience indicates that allergy and food intolerance is the most common trigger of bed-wetting. It is often an overlooked area as it is difficult to demonstrate by objective testing. However, offending foods can cause swelling of the mucosal lining of the bladder, which decreases the internal size or capacity of the bladder. This functional decrease in capacity is only apparent during the times that the offending food is eaten. The overall size of the bladder remains normal, with only the internal volume being decreased. In addition, swelling of the mucosal and muscle layers of the bladder reduces the ability of the bladder to stretch. The internal and external sphincters (valves) of the bladder are also subject to swelling as an allergic response. The usual result is that they are unable to contract tightly and may fatigue more quickly. In the presence of bladder edema, neurologic stimulus is probably more difficult to interpret.

### Case Study: *Nichole*

Nichole, age eight, was having problems with chronic bed-wetting which was still almost a nightly occurrence. This condition was creating a social problem for her as she had reached an age where she wanted to sleep over at her friends' houses, but didn't dare because of the bed-wetting. Her mother had tried everything she could think of to help Nichole. She had taken Nichole to her medical doctor for tests, but had been told that everything was normal.

Testing revealed that Nichole was intolerant to sugar, wheat, beef and mold. She was not digesting her food well. She was also nutrient deficient in vitamins A, C and E and iron.

The offending foods were removed from the diet. Nichole was given a nutrient supplement and plant enzymes to take at each meal, and an herbal extract to speed up healing of the lining of the intestinal tract. She received chiropractic adjustments directed at improving nerve and body function.

The bed-wetting began to improve by the second week of treatment and had completely ceased by the second month. Nichole showed a lot of motivation to get well as she had been very embarrassed by the bed-wetting. She followed her diet strictly at first. In Nichole's case sugar appeared to be the trigger that caused the symptoms. She soon found that she could eat almost anything except sugar. On occasion when she drank soda pop, she would have a wet night. Even this disappeared after eight months. Easter came along at this time, and Nichole ate a lot of chocolate Easter eggs. However, this time she did not wet the bed. She found that when she kept consumption of sugar occasional, she no longer wet the bed. She was able to eat all food groups without symptoms. Nichole remained free of bed-wetting.

The most common food identified as triggering bed-wetting is milk or dairy products, although it is possible for any food, combination of foods, or food groups to be responsible. Complete elimination of the offending foods is necessary during treatment. Concentrated plant enzymes should be given at each meal, with the dosage depending on the body size of the child. Yeast overgrowth or local infection of the urethra is common in many children with nocturnal enuresis (bedwetting). A good percentage of these children have a case history of recurrent middle ear infection and have been treated repeatedly with antibiotics. Local genital itchiness, allergies, eczema and ear infections are all symptomatic of yeast infection in children. *Lactobacillus acidophilus* and *bifidus* can be given to the child along with abstinence from the offending foods, especially dairy products.

Peanuts are frequent offenders, as are refined sugar products and wheat products such as bread and cereal.

Blood sugar imbalance is commonly associated with bed-wetting. However, sugar is not the only problem food here. Any food that reacts allergically can cause changes in blood sugar and lead to bed-wetting.

## Hyperactivity

Many of the same factors that create colic, ear infection and bed-wetting also create hyperactivity, short attention span and behavior and learning problems. The major areas to address are:

1. Poor nutrition and faulty digestion.
2. Food allergies and intolerance.
3. Environmental toxins.
4. Yeast overgrowth and parasites.
5. Repeated antibiotics and other medications.

All of the above can adversely affect a child's nervous system.

Children with ear infection due to allergic reactions often become those who are hyperactive and exhibit attention span deficits. They are the children receiving repeated doses of antibiotics that lead to yeast overgrowth, which in turn produces a "leaky" gut allowing allergy to emerge and weaken the immune system. This creates toxins which irritate the nervous system. With hyperactivity, elimination of allergens in the diet and the addition of plant enzyme therapy is a vital step.

# 15

# Additives Add Up to Allergy

There is only one thing to say about food additives: none of them do your health any good. Most of them either cause or have the potential to cause toxic and allergic reactions. The body reacts to foreign substances, and today we are seeing more and more occurrence of both additives and allergies.

Consider this:

1. Two and a half billion pounds of pesticides are released into the environment each year. Sixty percent of these pesticides are used by farmers.

2. Over 4,000 varieties of drugs are fed to animals which produce milk, eggs and meat. About half of all the drugs manufactured in the United States are given to farm animals, many of them as medicated feed.

Pesticide and drug residues in food are common. Food additives are substances, whether natural or synthetic, which are added to original food substances. Since almost every food in a can, bottle or package contains additives, we can see that over 90 percent of foods in the supermarket contain additives. All additives are potentially capable of causing allergic reactions. Over 6,000 different chemicals are available to be used in food manufacturing today. Most of these have become available in the last 45 years. Each person consumes five pounds of food additives per year. Since World War II, consumption of chemically altered foods has risen from 10 to 80 percent of the total diet. Since the ingestion of these chemicals and additives is a relatively new phenomenon, it appears certain that we are demanding that our bodies adapt to such offensive changes at too rapid a pace. There is little evidence to indicate that sufficient enzymes are manufactured by the body to metabolize these chemicals. When substances cannot be metabolized efficiently, they place stress on the body in the form of toxicity, leading to negative reactions. Some of the toxic effects of these additives are known. The consumer, whether suffering from allergies or any other health problem, should be aware of these negative effects.

## The Big Four

**1. Sulfites** come in many forms – sodium bisulfate and sodium or potassium metabisulfite, sulfur dioxide, sodium sulfite, potassium sulfite and bisulfate. Sulfites are used as preservatives and antioxidants. They keep fresh food from turning brown. Because allergy sufferers and asthmatics are particularly sensitive to them and because they have led to seventeen confirmed deaths in the United States, some laws have been passed limiting their use. However, sulfites are still allowed in many products. The most common products are wine, beer, fresh vegetables and fruit, citrus drinks, potato products such as chips and fries, fish and shrimp, dried fruits, fruit snacks and many frozen items such as potato products and TV dinners.

Hundreds of medications contain sulfites. It is ironic that while asthmatics are particularly sensitive to sulfites, many bronchodilators contain up to 6ppm (parts per million) of sulfur dioxide. When inhaled, this is enough to cause bronchospasm. Other drugs that contain sulfites include heart medications, steroids, antibiotics, pain medicines and muscle relaxants.

The average daily intake of sulfites with food eaten at home is 2 to 3 mg per day. In contrast, the average restaurant meal contains an estimated 25 to 200 mg of sulfites. In addition to their allergenic potential, sulfites destroy vitamin $B_1$ in foods.

**2. Tartrazine or Yellow Dye #5:** Most food dyes are known carcinogens. They are also potential allergens. Tartrazine imparts a yellow color to food. Several tons of food dyes are consumed every year. The chemical structure of Yellow Dye #5 is nearly identical to that of aspirin. People who are allergic to aspirin may also be allergic to this dye.

Soft drinks, candy and desserts are particularly high in tartrazine. About 500 drugs contain this dye as a coloring agent. The estimated average intake is 15 mg per day. However, some individuals or children consuming excess soft drinks and candy have intakes up to 150 mg per day. Tartrazine is a causative agent in bronchial asthma. Other common foods which contain this dye are cheese, cake mixes, frostings, canned vegetables, chewing gum, fruit juices, macaroni and cheese, meat tenderizer, puddings, salad dressings, ketchup, pickles, relishes, canned fruit, butter, margarine, baked goods, popsicles, fruit drinks, gelatins, colored cereals, banana and lime flavoring, mustards and wine coolers.

**3. BHA and BHT:** These preservatives and antioxidants were designed for use in petroleum products and rubber, but found their way into breakfast cereals. BHA and BHT can affect the nervous system and are known to cause behavioral problems in children. At levels now permitted in foods, there is evidence that BHT may convert hormones and oral contraceptives into carcinogenic agents. BHT has been banned from all foods in England.

People with urticaria (hives) and asthma often react allergically to BHA and BHT. Common foods that contain these chemicals are cereals, instant potato flakes, frozen dinners, baked goods, fruit drinks and many others.

**4. MSG:** Monosodium glutamate has an interesting history. Its usefulness as a flavor enhancer of foods is unequaled by any other additive. On the other hand, it is associated with a long list of negative health effects. A few years ago, MSG was removed from baby food because it was shown to cause damage to the brain stem in infants. If it is capable of this, what is it doing to everyone else, and why is it still found in so many foods? MSG masquerades under the names of "hydrolyzed vegetable protein," "autolysed yeast," "hydrolyzed yeast," "vegetable powder," or "natural flavors." If you read labels, you'll find that almost all packaged goods contain MSG in one form or another.

MSG occurs in larger amounts in foods than other additives, often in gram amounts rather than milligrams. The average daily intake is 1 gram. A typical Chinese meal contains 5 to 10 g MSG. Although MSG is ordinarily associated with Chinese food, nearly all restaurants use MSG. Below are some interesting facts about monosodium glutamate.

Over 20 million people in the United States are highly sensitive to MSG. If the dose is high enough, everyone will react to MSG.

Children are very sensitive to MSG. Exposure over time can result in behavioral disorders or impaired intellect. Brain damage is possible with prolonged exposure to high enough dosages.

Common symptoms of MSG usage include headache, asthma and chest pains. Other symptoms are diarrhea, blurred vision, fatigue, hot flashes, numbness around the face, sweating, palpitations and urinary discomfort.

Fast food restaurants are particularly heavy users of MSG. Practically everything that is breaded contains MSG. This includes fried chicken and chicken nuggets, fried fish, cheese balls and sticks, fried zucchini, onion rings and breaded meats such as pork chops and veal Parmesan. The product "Accent" is pure MSG. Who would suspect that MSG may be added to some brands of "water packed" tuna or dry roasted nuts? Soy sauce, bouillon and canned and dry soups are more obvious sources. Other foods commonly containing MSG are ketchup, frozen dinners, frozen vegetables, canned and cured meats and noodle dishes.

Vitamin $B_6$ is necessary for the metabolism of MSG. Therefore, MSG has the effect of causing vitamin $B_6$ deficiency. $B_6$ in sufficient quantities has been known to stop reactions to MSG.

## Other Additives

While the additives already mentioned are especially important to individuals with allergy, there are other additives used in food that deserve attention.

**Nitrates and Nitrites:** These are used primarily as preservatives in meats. They give a pink color to cured meat such as lunch meats, hot dogs, bacon, ham and sausages. Nitrites combine with stomach fluids to form nitrosamines, powerful cancer-causing agents.

**Aspartame:** More lawsuits have been launched against Aspartame in the length of time it has been on the market than any other artificial sweetener. It was first approved for use in 1981. By 1985, more than 800 million pounds were used each year in the United States. Possible symptoms include headaches, dizziness, behavioral changes, convulsions, diarrhea and memory loss. Recognized allergic symptoms are severe itching, hives and swelling of the lips, mouth, tongue and throat. Studies show that a high intake of Aspartame could cause brain damage in infants. For this reason, some obstetricians advise mothers not to consume products with Aspartame during pregnancy or breast feeding. Common products containing Aspartame are many diet foods, gelatins, soft drinks, fruit drink mixes and Equal.

**Benzoic Acid and Sodium Benzoate:** These additives are used as preservatives and anti-fungal agents. They affect the nervous system and are involved in allergic reactions such as asthma, stomach irritations and hyperactivity in children.

**EDTA:** EDTA has the ability to bind with metal particles and remove them from the body. However, during this process, it also removes essential metals such as iron and zinc. Foods which contain EDTA include margarine, salad dressings, frozen dinners and many others.

**Propyl Gallate:** This additive is known to precipitate allergic and asthmatic reactions. It is found in frozen dinners, gravy mixes, turkey sausage and other products. It is used as an antioxidant to keep fats from becoming rancid.

**Alginates:** Many forms of alginate are used in processed foods. There is ammonium, calcium, potassium, sodium and glycol alginate, and there are also algin derivatives. Alginates stabilize and impart a creamy texture to foods such as ice cream, salad dressings, cheese spreads and frozen dinners. Alginates are being tested in relation to reproductive problems.

**Artificial Flavors:** Approximately 1,500 artificial flavors are used in food production. Common flavors are butyl acetate, benzaldehyde, methyl salicylates and benzyl alcohol. They are best known to cause hyperactivity in children, although depression and reproductive problems have also been associated with them.

**Bromate:** Calcium bromate and potassium bromate are used as dough conditioners. Therefore, they are found primarily in baked goods and bread, bread crumbs and refrigerated dough. Bromates are very toxic in high doses.

## Alcohol

Alcohol contributes to food allergy in several ways:

It increases intestinal permeability, thereby allowing potential allergenic substances to be absorbed into the blood stream and precipitate reactions. It is a major contributor to the "leaky gut" syndrome.

Alcohol is very rapidly absorbed from the stomach and intestine. This rapid absorption, coupled with the fact that alcohol carries with it the reactivity of the food from which it was made, makes it a potent allergen. This is what makes it a powerful addictant, which we commonly observe as alcoholism. For example, in clinical studies, social drinkers who become inebriated on as little as two drinks of beer or whisky were found to be sensitive to corn, wheat, malt, barley, rye or yeast. Most alcoholic beverages are not required to carry on their labels a list of the ingredients, making it difficult for the consumer to know what they contain, or from what they were made.

Corn, barley, rye, wheat, oats and rice are the common grains used in the production of straight and blended whisky and vodka. The first three are generally used to make gin. Corn and barley are the usual grains used in beer and ale. Other ingredients in alcoholic beverages such as cane sugar, malt or yeast can also produce allergic reactions. If a person is allergic to the grain from which the alcohol was made, the reaction can be exaggerated or more extreme than a reaction to the grain itself due to the rapid absorption of the alcohol.

Some people react to the pesticide residues contained in the beverage. Pesticides, such as the chlorinated hydrocarbons which came into use after 1945, can cause symptoms such as redness in the face, hyperactivity, headache and depression. In addition to the fact that alcohol is absorbed rapidly, it tends to cause more rapid absorption of some foods.

When alcoholics stop drinking, they tend to substitute the edible form of their specific addictants. Most alcoholics are allergic to corn.

When they stop drinking, they substitute corn sugar found in candy, cookies and doughnuts or other products containing corn sugar, dextrose or glucose. This continues both the addiction and the craving. Anything that weakens the intestinal membranes, making them more permeable, leads to increased susceptibility to allergy. Many common drugs other than alcohol do this. Heavy or prolonged drug usage especially can damage the intestines and lead to increased permeability. Some of the common drugs involved are:

| | | |
|---|---|---|
| Aspirin, | Coumadin | Motrin or |
| Bufferin, | Dolobid | Ibuprofen |
| Excedrin | Fiorinal | Naprosyn |
| Butazoladin | Fenoprin | Tanderil |
| Clinoril | Heparin | Tolectin |
| cortisone | Indocin | |

# 16

# Body, Mind and Allergy

We often hear these days of the body-mind connection: the idea that thoughts can control certain internal functions of the body. We hear stories of Eastern masters who appear to have achieved mental control over such body functions as blood pressure, heartbeat and respiration. The discovery of biofeedback around 1958 piqued many western scientists' curiosity about how the mind can control specific body functions. Using various machines, biofeedback can monitor minute changes in body functions that previously were believed to be beyond conscious control. Biofeedback is also used to increase awareness of the link between the body and the mind. With biofeedback, patients have been taught how to voluntarily control heart rate, blood pressure, muscular tension, anxiety, headaches, insomnia and stomach acidity. Using similar techniques, some doctors have achieved good results in cancer patients by having the patient visualize little cells like Pac Man eating up cancer cells.

How do thoughts influence the body? While not all the mechanisms are known, some of the influencing pathways have been discovered. According to Dr. M.T. Morter, Jr., thoughts are energy. He explains, "By understanding that mental activity generates energy and that this energy is transformed into the energy fields of the body, we can understand why thoughts and the mind are so important in gaining, restoring, or maintaining physical health."

Scientist Cleve Backster pioneered research on the idea that there is electrical activity at the cellular level and that this electrical activity can be influenced by thoughts. Using human cells that he had scraped from the roof of the mouth, Backster perfected a method of electroding them so they could be monitored with electroencephalogram-type instruments measuring their net electrical potential. Backster then demonstrated that these cells were capable of reacting when the donor was emotionally stressed. In one case, a female donor of mouth cells reacted emotionally when she watched circumstances leading to a rape scene on television. Even though her mouth cells were being monitored half a mile away, the cells reacted with sharp swings on the recording graph at the exact time of the rape scene. In another example, a male donor was asked to watch a war scene while his mouth cells were being monitored. As he emotionally reacted to the scene of a plane crash, his mouth cells recorded a change on the recording graph.

If emotionally charged thoughts are capable of changing electrical impulses of cells which are located half a mile away from the body, thoughts are certainly capable of influencing cells still located in the body.

Thoughts can be generated by external or internal stimuli. If we could shrink down to the size of an atom residing in the brain, we might observe something like this: in simplified form, thought generation is believed to occur when electrons change orbit. The body is made up of atoms. Atoms contain both electrons and protons with negative and positive charges. The electrons revolve within the atom in spatial domains known as orbitals. Each orbital possesses a specific frequency and energetic characteristics. When energy of a specific frequency (a stimulus) is delivered to the electron, it will excite or "boost" it into the next highest orbital. When this occurs with enough electrons, a thought may be created or intensified.

It is truly exciting to discover that by using the conscious mind, you can "give birth" to thousands of thoughts each day and even direct them to do your bidding! The fact that thoughts can carry out your intent makes it doubly important that you focus your thoughts on only the things that you want. If you want a healthy body, it is necessary that only health-building thoughts be generated.

Once generated, where do the thoughts go? Through Backster's experiments, it appears that some of the thoughts remain on the energetic level influencing the body's cells. Some thought energy takes other routes.

Guyton's *Textbook of Medical Physiology* tells us that, "When a person experiences some powerful depressing or exciting thought, a portion of the signal is transmitted into the hypothalamus." The hypothalamus is comprised of neurological tissue lying at the lower portion of the brain. It is so small it composes less than one percent of the total brain mass, yet it is responsible for an immense number of vital body functions. The hypothalamus influences the heart rate, arterial blood pressure, body temperature, thirst, hunger and satiety, uterine contractions and water excretion. It also controls the pituitary gland, known as the "master gland" of the body, releasing hormones into the blood stream in response to stimuli. Thoughts can be translated into numerous neurological and hormonal stimuli which can reach any part of the body. In the past, most of these functions have been considered to be "autonomic" or taking place without conscious control.

The hypothalamus, once thought to be a gland, is actually a tiny extension of the brain which has one very unique characteristic. It is the only part of the brain that has direct blood contact. The rest of the brain and the bones of the skull have protective membranes called the blood-brain barrier. A series of transport mechanisms in this membrane protect the brain from small variations in the composition of the blood. For example, large protein particles cannot enter the brain but proteins in the form of amino acids can. The transport mechanisms select what can enter the brain and what cannot. Alcohol and steroid hormones readily penetrate the blood-brain barrier.

The hypothalamus, however, deals directly with the blood and all its constituents. It acts like a thermostat taking information from the blood and secreting hormones in response. What stimulates the hypothalamus is *what is in the blood*. What is in the blood depends largely on what you eat and how well you digest and absorb it. It is not specifically known what adverse effects undigested particles of food, residues of drugs or chemicals, or inflammatory products of allergic reactions, such as histamine, have on the hypothalamus. However, it seems apparent that if abnormal particles reach this area through the blood, an alarm response of the hypothalamus will send signals to the rest of the body that may not be in the interest of health. Altered information in means altered information out.

Guyton states in the *Textbook of Medical Physiology,* "Even the concentrations of nutrients, electrolytes, water and various hormones in the blood excite or inhibit various portions of the hypothalamus. Thus, the hypothalamus is a collecting center for information conveyed with the internal well-being of the body."

Where does this information sent by the hypothalamus go? Most of it goes straight to the pituitary gland. Nearly all of the pituitary secretions are controlled either by hormone stimulation or nerve stimulation from the hypothalamus. The anterior pituitary is controlled by hormones arriving through blood vessels, and the posterior pituitary is controlled by nerve fibers from the hypothalamus. Nerve signals reach the hypothalamus from nearly all possible sources in the nervous system. With a direct blood vessel connection and a direct nerve connection to the pituitary, the entire body is thus influenced. With portions of thought signals being directed through the hypothalamus, we have a real physical body-mind connection.

The functions in the body occur, for the most part, without your conscious thought. However, you do have control over the basic mechanism by what you give the hypothalamus to evaluate. The majority of stimuli reach the hypothalamus as an end result of what you eat, drink and think.

Since food is the largest single stimulus to the body on a daily basis, let's look more closely at the role it plays. Once food is eaten, the body must process it through a series of enzyme reactions. Like all functions of the body, the ability to produce enzymes is not inexhaustible. Researchers think that it takes several generations to build enzymes for a new food. This means when an entirely new food is eaten, the body may not have enzymes to digest it properly. After several generations of eating this food, the body eventually adapts and produces the enzymes to deal with it. In the meantime, the preceding generations have stressed their enzyme systems with unknown negative effects on their health.

156

It has been estimated that because of the refining and processing of food, the majority of food eaten today is new since the 1940s. No one knows what enzymes are necessary to break down the various chemicals used in processed foods to enhance their appearance and extend their shelf life. It is likely that we have not built enzyme systems to deal with these foods yet. Possibly the chemicals deplete our enzymes at a faster rate than eating a food in the natural state. If these foods are not broken down sufficiently in the digestive tract, what signals are they conveying through the blood stream to the hypothalamus which in turn controls nearly all our body processes? These are questions that have not been answered to date.

Zane R. Gard, MD expressed his views on this matter in the April 1987 issue of the *Townsend Letter:* "Three thousand [chemicals] have been identified as intentionally added to food supplies and over 700 in drinking water. During food processing and storage more than 10,000 other compounds can become an integral part of many commonly used foods." And this is just in foods. What about all the thousands of chemicals released into the environment every year? All of these tend to work their way back into the human body. More than 6,000 new chemicals are tested in the United States each week. Over 7,000,000 distinct chemical compounds have appeared in scientific literature since 1965. Once in the body, enzymes must break down all these chemical compounds. There is no scientific proof to date that the body is capable of building enzymes to do the job. Through this one mechanism, the ingestion and subsequent breakdown of foods and chemicals that in turn are conveyed through the blood stream to the hypothalamus, our bodies and minds either reap the rewards of the beneficial nutrients supplied or the damage caused by the combined effects of toxic chemicals and lack of nutrients in processed foods.

# 17

# Energy Allergy – A New Frontier

Probably the most fascinating and controversial subject relating to health today is in the realm of energy. Exploring the energy of the body can be considered an exciting new frontier as we strive to learn more about its properties and how to use them to help maintain and restore health. However, the emergence of a new "energy" medicine is not without problems. Many doctors regard it as incompatible with existing medical opinion. Why should this be? Robert O. Becker, MD explains the differing philosophies in his book *Cross Currents:* "The proponents of orthodox medicine – the kind taught in medical schools and promoted by the Medical Association (AMA) and the Food and Drug Administration (FDA) – are absolutely convinced that the body is simply a machine that cannot heal itself, and the only appropriate therapies are powerful drugs and mechanical technologies. Proponents of "energy" medicine, on the other hand, believe that the body is more than a machine, and that it is capable not only of healing itself but also of performing other actions that lie completely outside the realm of established science. The latter practitioners believe that an appropriate therapy is one that either encourages the body's own energetic systems or that adds external energy to those systems."

Alongside this divergence of opinion within the medical establishment, doctors in many parts of the world have gone ahead with measuring electrical currents and studying the electrical fields of the body.

Much of this work has been done in Russia and to a lesser extent elsewhere in Europe. Because of recently developed instruments, Western scientists are becoming more involved in research of this type. Through this research, it has been discovered that the body has both electrical and magnetic properties.

Energy of the body has been described for thousands of years by the Chinese who call it "Chi" and the Hindus who call it "Prana." We sometimes refer to it as the "vital force" or "life force." Acupuncture works on the energy fields of the body by attempting to balance them. Energy is believed to flow along energy pathways of the body, called meridians. Using modern instruments, scientists have been able to confirm the existence of meridians – by measuring them with sensitive electronic instruments and tracing them using radioactive isotopes.

The voltmeter was an early instrument used to measure the force field of the body. Using this instrument, the force field was found to extend beyond the surface of the skin: it was measured through electrodes held a short distance from the skin and not in contact with it. Since the voltmeter required virtually no current for its operation, this indicated that an actual field was being measured.

You are probably familiar with modern diagnostic machines that measure electrical impulses. The electrocardiogram measures electrical impulses of the heart and the electroencephalogram measures electrical waves and activity of the brain.

In his book *Blueprint for Immortality* Harold Saxton Burr writes, "There are electrical properties wherever there is life." Robert O. Becker, MD states, "Drawing upon the concepts of information theory and solid state physics, and aided by instruments of vastly improved sensitivity and sophistication, we have described electronic controlled systems within the body that regulate such functions as growth and healing, and that also serve as the substrate for our internal control and communication systems."

The body is made up of atoms with positive and negative charges in motion. Physics tells us that any time there is a flow of electrons, a magnetic field will be produced in the space around it. Using this law, the motion of ions (atoms with a positive or negative charge) inside the body would generate weak magnetic fields. This can be illustrated by the flow of electric currents in the brain which produces a magnetic field around the head. The development of the super-conducting quantum interference device (SQUID) around 1970 led to the discovery of this magnetic field in the space around the human head. The SQUID can measure the magnetic field from several feet away from the head! More recently, scientists have also been able to record the magnetic field associated with the nerve impulse itself.

An even more startling discovery demonstrates the magnetic nature of living organisms. A chain of tiny magnets inside a living bacterium has been seen under the electron microscope. These magnets are actually tiny crystals of magnetite, a natural magnetic mineral. We have long suspected that homing pigeons are able to derive directional information from the earth's magnetic field. Recently, Dr. Charles Walcott has discovered magnetite crystals on the surface of the pigeons' brains. These crystals appear to be connected to the brain by nerve fibers. In experiments in England, Dr. Robin Baker has tentatively located the corresponding magnetic area in humans. The location appears to be in the back wall of the ethmoid sinus of the skull.

It has been known that nerves transmit information throughout the body by electrical and chemical means. Hormones carry messages from one gland to another and to other parts of the body. Now we are beginning to see that electromagnetic waves also carry information capable of communicating between organs, tissues and cells. According to Dr. F.A. Popp, a German physician, the amount of information being transmitted per second by just one cell of the body is so great that it would take a hundred years to read it if it were printed. Dr. Popp has shown that "transmitters and receivers" exist in the double helix of the DNA of the cell nucleus.

He has further determined that electromagnetic waves, which move with the speed of light, are dependent upon the presence of protons, electrons and minerals. Dr. Becker backs up this idea. He writes, "Magnetic and electromagnetic fields have energy, can carry information, and are produced by electrical current."

Guyton's *Textbook of Medical Physiology* states, "Electrical potentials exist across the membranes of all cells of the body and some cells, such as nerve cells and muscle cells, are excitable, that is, capable of self-generation of electrochemical impulses at their membranes and in some instances, employment of these impulses to transmit signals along the membranes."

The brain shows continuous electrical activity. Brain waves, as recorded at the surface of the head, vary in intensity from zero to 300 millivolts. Their frequency range is from one cycle every several seconds to 50 or more cycles per second.

Let's stretch our imaginations and take a look at what Richard Gerber, MD has to say about the human body and its "energetic" properties. "We know through modern quantum physics that the physical body is actually a unique aggregation of physical particles of matter which, themselves, are points of frozen light. Interfaced with this physical body of light are additional light bodies composed of subtle energetic matter of higher frequency levels than that which the physical body can perceive."

Your body is constantly forming new cells to replace tired and worn out cells. The force that activates the formation and division of these new cells is believed to be magnetic energy. It now appears that biochemistry is controlled by the "bioenergy" of the body. This "bioenergy" was first captured on film by the Russian scientists, Semjon and Valentina Kirlian who used a special form of electrophotography. Their pictures showed a radiating luminescence around living organisms, including the human body. In further studies using this photographic method, these fields around the body are seen to fluctuate according to metabolic activities taking place inside the body. For example, when healthy individuals eat raw food, the field responds with vibrant intensity. When highly refined, processed food is eaten, the field becomes less vibrant.

Cells depend on magnetic energy to function properly. Cells make up the tissues that make up the organs and glands which require a constant presence of magnetic energy. The natural vibrational frequencies of the body are controlled by the positive and negative magnetic fields.

If there is an imbalance in electromagnetic radiation in an organ or tissue, function of that organ or tissue is disturbed. This disturbance is called "disease."

162

Many scientists now believe that disease, including allergy, can first be detected as a disturbance of the normal flow and balance of energy in the body. If this disturbance continues long enough, changes eventually manifest themselves in the physical tissues.

It appears that just as wrong food can lead to disease, so can wrong electromagnetic waves. Researchers have found that each organ in the body has its own electromagnetic wave frequency. If for any reason the electromagnetic waves are disturbed and the body is unable to correct the disturbance, the frequency of the waves is changed. If it remains changed for a long enough time, pathology develops in the tissues. In other words, abnormal waves develop when the normal waves are blocked or impeded.

The early symptoms of allergy often begin as small shifts in the pattern of the body's energy. Dr. Kenyon, in Liverpool, England, has studied this phenomenon for a number of years. He believes that the body can detect a harmful substance within its field and will react by producing minute changes in its electrical responses. Also, if an organ in the body is unhealthy, it is unable to maintain a normal supply of energy and its deficiency can be measured. According to Dr. Kenyon, allergy is primarily an electrical phenomenon, and if it continues long enough, it will eventually produce changes in the blood and other tissues.

Since every cell in the body produces energy and has a polarity, energy is the fundamental principle that underlies everything that happens in the body, including biochemical changes. If allergy is considered as an energy disturbance, it means that when allergy is present, the flow of energy is disturbed, unbalanced or blocked. The result is a biochemical process that cannot proceed as it otherwise might. The flow of energy in the body regulates and controls all body processes including the utilization of nutritional substances and the function of the immune system.

Research in biomagnetics has established that a proper balance between the positive and negative magnetic poles in the human body is necessary for health and life itself. Each cell in the body is itself a weak magnet with a positive and negative pole. If a balance is to be maintained between these poles, then we must ask the question, how do these electromagnetic poles become disturbed in humans?

It appears that some of the more common stressors are toxins and chemicals in the food and environment. These, along with allergens, nutritional deficiencies, bacterial and viral infections, all carry a positive magnetic charge that when prolonged can unbalance the positive and negative relationship necessary for health. These stressors may lead to magnetic energy imbalance which results in physical and emotional illnesses. Although less recognized, the amount of environmental radiation that the body is exposed to on a daily basis has become an increasingly common stressor. This environmental radiation is termed "electropollution" or "electromagnetic contamination."

The natural pulsing frequency of the earth has been determined to be about 7.9 cycles per second. This is also the healthy vibrational frequency of the human body as a whole. Individual organs have their individual frequencies. For instance, the frequency of the brain at rest has been determined to be 1 to 2 cycles per second; awake is 8 to 12 cycles per second; and during concentration is 18 to 22 cycles per second. The normal electromagnetic fields of the body are disturbed when the body is exposed over time to other frequencies.

Man-made radiation produces frequencies that are not found in nature, and which are not present in the normal electromagnetic spectrum of the earth. We are all aware that X-rays are damaging to human cells. X-rays are high frequency, ionizing radiation which can cause cancer and genetic changes. However, we are not so familiar with other forms of man-made radiation. We can't see, hear, taste or smell radiation, and consequently tend not to be aware of it. According to Dr. Robert O. Becker, we are now existing in a "world of energy," the majority of which is man-made radiation which has never before existed on the earth.

What are some common sources of this radiation? We may not think of televisions, stereos and computers as sources, but they do emit radiation. Other sources include fluorescent lights, electric calculators, microwave ovens, telephones, electric blankets, electric heaters, high voltage power lines, electronic security systems, electric clocks and automobiles with computerized equipment. Length of exposure is a critical factor: the longer the exposure, the more the potential harm. Appliances such as hand-held electric hair dryers and electric shavers provide short exposure, compared to constant exposure to high voltage power lines located near a home.

Dr. Becker writes in his book *Cross Currents,* "In addition, new technologies have appeared. Commercial telephone and television satellite transmitters and relays blanket the Earth from 25,000 miles out in space. Military satellites cruise by every point on Earth once an hour, and from their altitude of only 250 miles, they bounce radar beams off its surface to produce images for later 'downloading' over their home countries. New TV and FM stations come on the air weekly. The industry has placed in the hands of the public such gadgets as citizen-band radios and cellular telephones.

"Engineers propose gigantic solar-power stations in space, which would relay the electrical energy to Earth by means of enormously powerful microwave beams. Electrical power transmission lines are operating at millions of volts and thousands of amperes of current. Military services of every country use all parts of the electromagnetic spectrum for communications and surveillance, and the use of electromagnetic energy as an antipersonnel weapon is being studied."

Dr. Becker further states, "The scientific evidence leads to only one conclusion: that exposure of living organisms to abnormal electromagnetic fields results in significant abnormalities in physiology and function."

As little as 100 years ago, humans were exposed to only the Earth's magnetic field. Less than four generations later, there is bombardment of man-made radiation. So much so, that Dr. Becker feels "We have almost reached a state by which the entire electromagnetic spectrum has been filled up with man-made frequencies."

Electropollution is gaining recognition as a precipitator of many chronic degenerative diseases, including allergy. In fact, one aspect of this is the new condition called *electromagnetic hypersensitivity syndrome,* caused by living in an abnormal electromagnetic environment.

Dr. William Rae heads the Environmental Health Center in Dallas, Texas. Here he tests patients with neurological and allergic symptoms by exposing them to a spectrum of electromagnetic fields. This testing is accomplished without the patients' conscious awareness. Dr. Rae finds a consistent sensitivity to specific frequencies in most patients he tests, thereby establishing that electromagnetic hypersensitivity is a real clinical entity.

Symptoms that have been found in association with electromagnetic hypersensitivity syndrome include:

| | |
|---|---|
| chronic fatigue | confusion |
| inability to concentrate | depression |
| sleep disturbances | poor memory |
| flu-like conditions | mood swings |
| abnormal behavior | irritability |
| skin eruptions | muscular weakness |
| muscle and heart pain | |

Other evidence that man-made radiation affects human physiology and function is seen in the following examples. Microwave radiation exposure has been linked to cataract formation. Parts of the body especially vulnerable to microwave radiation are the eye, gallbladder, digestive tract and testes. Dr. Becker states that all microwave ovens emit an average of 120 microwatts near the door.

Reports of the hazard of living near high tension power lines have been creeping in for more than twenty years. One of the most famous studies ever done on the relationship of childhood leukemia and the effects of the high tension power lines appeared in the *New Yorker* magazine in June, 1989. The study cited a two- to three-fold increase in leukemia rates for children who lived in homes near high current lines.

Other adverse biological effects have been reported. Dr. John Ott discovered that red blood cells clump together when in close proximity to a video display terminal. Video display terminals have also been linked to conditions such as altered cell growth, altered metabolism of protein, carbohydrates and fats, increased cancers and leukemia and miscarriages.

A New York study in 1987 demonstrated that exposure to power lines and radiation from household appliances can increase the rate at which cancer cells grow and can produce long-lasting behavior alterations and changes in brain neurotransmitters.

Dr. Daniel B. Lyle of Loma Linda, California, reported that exposure of human T-cell lymphocytes (the immune system's killer cells) to a 60 Hz electric field for 48 hours significantly reduced their ability to fight foreign invaders. This is evidence of a direct link between common electrical fields and the immune system.

There is also evidence that low frequency fields interfere with the rate at which cells release and absorb calcium. Dr. Ross Adey concludes that low frequency electromagnetic fields can jam the communication signals between cells.

It is important to become aware of the sources and cumulative effects of radiation exposure, particularly if your body is already compromised and exhibiting signs of chronic disease or allergy. Limiting sources of pollution of all types helps increase the immune system's power to combat illness. While you cannot eliminate all the sources of electropollution in today's world, you can limit your exposure. Some of the things you can do in your immediate environment are:

1. Sit at least four to six feet from the television set and limit time in front of it.
2. Limit your exposure around microwave ovens, or do not use them. Do not let children stand and watch food cook.
3. Obtain full spectrum lighting for fluorescent lights. Russian scientists report that the body's tolerance to environmental pollutants is increased by full spectrum lights.
4. Avoid buying a home near high tension power lines or a microwave tower.
5. Do not use an electric blanket, or turn it off while occupying the bed.
6. Do not use a waterbed, or turn off the heater while occupying the bed.
7. Move digital alarm clocks and radios at least three feet away from the bed.
8. Buy cars without computer components.
9. Use a VDT screen for your computer to help block radiation.
10. Discuss radiation exposure with your doctor prior to having diagnostic X-rays taken. Request the minimum number of views necessary.
11. Avoid living near a nuclear power station, or next to a nuclear disposal site.

12. Avoid products containing radio-luminous dials and markers.
13. Some eyeglass lenses may contain uranium or thorium to enhance optical quality. Studies show these eyeglasses emit one millirad an hour.

Exposure to radiation from any source is an additional stressor to the body, especially to its electromagnetic fields. It is best to limit exposure by becoming aware of the possible sources of radiation in the environment. By removing unnecessary stressors from the environment, a person suffering from allergic problems will respond to treatment more rapidly.

# 18

## Seven Steps to Health

This chapter is not designed for self treatment. It is included for information only, to enable you to understand the steps necessary for recovery from allergy and allergic disorders. Understanding the process allows you to take a more active role in your healing and make informed decisions concerning your care.

Again, the following information, presented in seven steps, is for educational purposes only. It is not a recommendation for treatment.

Genetics, stress and emotions have traditionally been catch-alls for the cause of allergy. It is now apparent that allergy is the result of toxicity from all sources, and deficiencies, primarily of enzymes, vitamins and minerals. Environmental triggers of allergic episodes are vastly under-recognized.

The Pottenger cat studies clearly demonstrate that allergy can be produced at will through diet in one to three generations of cats, and also reversed in one to three generations of cats through improved diet. Poor digestion of food is a precursor to a great deal of allergy. How do so many people get a compromised digestive tract? By putting too much processed, heat-treated and chemicalized food into the system when no proof exists that humans are able to digest it. Therefore, the body must make changes and adaptations in order to survive.

Most books on allergy advise an elimination diet, in which you eliminate the allergenic foods for months or years. Other books encourage you to become a "super sleuth" tracking down "hidden food allergies" looking for undetectable fragments of chemicals and ingredients which can be hidden in your meals, your house or your environment. Still other books recommend that you rotate your foods, eating the same food only once every four to five days, or keeping a diet diary of everything you eat. While all these are good advice and help to control allergies, they do not get you well permanently. They are good methods as long as you continue to follow them.

There are other, more effective approaches to the allergy problem. When you have allergies, you have enzyme deficiency, energy imbalance or both. The amount of treatment required to reverse these conditions depends on the type of allergy, its severity and duration and the strength of the body's immune system. Four to six weeks is an average treatment time required to turn the disease process around and allow for tissue healing. Persons with mild allergic conditions respond faster than those with severe symptoms. This is because the treatment process must be administered more slowly in acutely ill persons. Following is a basic program that has worked with wonderful success on thousands of patients.

The seven healing steps are:
1. Prepare the body to get well.
2. Eliminate allergens.
3. Enzyme therapy.
4. Build the immune system.
5. Professional care.
6. Healing techniques and dietary follow-up.
7. Think wellness and wholeness.

## Step One:
### *Prepare the body to get well.*

Preparing the body means lowering the allergic or toxic load. Check your environment and eliminate sources of toxins, molds and fungi. Inspect gas stoves and furnaces to ensure there are no fumes or leaks. Use earth-friendly, less toxic household cleaners, cosmetics and personal care products. Avoid exposure to radiation.

Obtain a pure, clean source of water. Tap water is not recommended. Reverse osmosis or distilled water is preferable. The quality of bottled water can be difficult to determine. Before drinking bottled water, you should check with the company as to source of the water, content and quality.

Next, it is helpful to clean out the body. A fresh fruit and vegetable juice diet for three to ten days is desirable. This juice diet is not absolutely essential to the program, but it does lower the toxic load of the body and speeds up the healing process. It requires that you obtain a good juicer and use only fresh, preferably organically-grown, raw fruits and vegetables. Health food stores carry good books on how to prepare juice, complete with many juice recipes.

A big source of toxicity is infection by invading organisms: yeasts, fungi and parasites. Allergic individuals tend to have a high incidence of such infections, as they underlie the allergic condition. The organisms constitute a major source of toxicity and stress to the immune system, while the victim is often unaware of their presence. In order to regain health, these infections and infestations, if present, must be recognized and brought under control.

Candidiasis has come to the forefront because of increased publicity in recent years. It is more likely to be recognized than other infestations or infections by organisms. Many parasites are cyclic, going through dormant and active phases, which means that they cannot always be found by testing. If suspected, the tests should be performed several times in order to rule out the presence of these organisms.

There are many good therapies for candidiasis. Some programs, however, work faster than others and some are only temporarily effective. It is not uncommon for the afflicted individual to be on a "Candida diet" for months and still not be restored to health. Another problem commonly seen is the removal of foods from the diet for such a lengthy time that the body 's nutritional state can be compromised. In some cases, the patient becomes anxious and fanatical about foods in general – another undesirable state. These extremes are not necessary, even in the severest cases. A lack of understanding about the objectives to be reached is usually at the root of the problem.

A sensible program of diet, nutrients and an understanding of the goals will bring Candida under control in a short time. Since Candida is a normal inhabitant of the intestine, the goal is not to kill it off completely. The goal is to bring its numbers back in balance with the other normal residents of the colon, and then to keep them in line by increasing the general health of the person and his immune system.

The following program has proven successful because it is quickly effective without being overly restrictive, which leads to excellent patient compliance. In order to diminish the number of Candida organisms, a formula similar to this can be used:

| | |
|---|---|
| vitamin E | 5 IU |
| biotin | 50 mcg |
| calcium | 30 mg |
| magnesium | 25 mg |
| potassium | 30 mg |
| special base of caprylic acid | 300 mg |
| propionic acid | 100 mg |
| sorbic acid | 100 mg |

Three capsules a day taken morning, noon and night until the bottle is gone is generally all that is required. At the same time, a good quality *Lactobacillus acidophilus* supplement should be taken. Quality products can be found in the refrigerated portion of the health food store.

When a formula such as the above is used, the diet does not have to be unduly strict. Only the worst offending foods are eliminated and only for four weeks. Almost everyone will respond in this period of time. If a person does not respond, either the products chosen are not of good quality or the person is not following the program for the prescribed time.

A sample diet for the Candida patient will look like this:
Eliminate from the diet:
all refined sugar and sugar products (read labels for listing of glucose, dextrose, etc.)
breads that contain yeast
cheese
mushrooms
refined and processed foods that list yeast on the label

Foods that may be eaten:
  all fresh vegetables and fruits
  whole grains and unleavened breads
  nuts and seeds
  all fresh meats if desired
  butter, no margarine
  fresh fruit juice if it is diluted in half with water
  pure maple syrup in very small quantities (1 tbsp. per day or less)
    may be used for a sweetener.

Sweets feed the Candida organism, so it is wise not to overdo fruits or fruit juices or the maple syrup. Yeast products often react allergically in the body when Candida is present, which is why exclusion of all yeast products is necessary.

Drink six to eight glasses of pure water per day. There will be toxicity as the Candida breaks down and is eliminated. The water will dilute the toxins, preventing discomforts that might otherwise occur. Symptoms that indicate you are not drinking enough water at this time include headaches, chills, fever, muscle aches, nausea and rashes. This program will work for almost all yeasts and fungi.

When parasites are present, herbal formulas will help to eliminate them. Formulas containing black walnut, pumpkin seeds, *Artemisia annua* and garlic have been effective. Use a formula of several herbs. This formula should be taken morning and night for five days, discontinued for three days, then repeated morning and night continuing this schedule. This helps interrupt the life cycle of the parasite from its cyst (dormant) stage to its larva (active) stage.

A herbal formula that is extremely helpful for healing the lining of the digestive tract is a liquid containing artichoke, dandelion and ten other herbs. It will produce noticeable healing changes very rapidly, usually within three days. The ten other herbs are turmeric root, St. Mary's thistle, blessed thistle, buckbean leaves, milfoil herb, gentian root, wormwood, calamus root, camomile and fennel. Good quality liquid chlorophyll is also beneficial.

A complete program consists of the following:
  1. Taking herbal and nutrient formulas to either diminish the number or kill off the pathogenic organisms.

2. Reculturing the bowel.

3. Repairing tissues.

When organisms such as Candida and other parasites are eliminated or brought under control, it is not unusual for 80 percent of the allergies displayed by the patient to be improved. This would be after just four weeks on the above program.

Limiting toxicity from the environment, food, water and pathological organisms is the first step to getting well. These conditions are not present in all allergic individuals, but when they do exist they must be addressed or wellness from allergies will not result.

## Step Two:
### *Eliminate allergens.*

Eliminate the main food allergens for the first four weeks. If you do not know to what you are allergic, you have two choices:

1. Eliminate the most common allergens such as dairy products, especially milk and cheese, wheat, eggs, corn and pork and all obvious chemicals in your environment.

2. Consult one of the doctors from the referral directory in the "Resources" section of this book.

On an effective program, foods are temporarily eliminated in order to give the digestive and immune systems time to recover and heal. After four weeks the foods can be reintroduced one at a time, if they are foods recommended for health. If they are destructive foods such as homogenized, pasteurized milk or potato chips, they should not be reintroduced.

## Step Three:
### *Enzyme therapy.*

Enzyme therapy is the cornerstone of effective allergy treatment. This safe and non-toxic therapy has one major advantage: it has the power to eliminate allergies.

In the clinical setting plant enzymes have proven to be a quick and efficient way to restore health from allergies. For our purposes, there are three categories of therapeutic enzymes: plant enymes, pancreatic enzymes, and antioxidant enzymes.

**Plant enzymes:** These are enzymes taken from plants under low heat conditions and concentrated. They contain protease, amylase, lipase and cellulase. They are the only enzymes capable of working both in the stomach and the small intestine as they are active at a pH range of approximately 3 to 9. After ingestion of food, they help the digestive process for up to an hour before the stomach pH finally falls below 3. Later, they are reactivated in the alkaline pH of the small intestine and help to complete the process of digestion.

When plant enzymes are given between meals, instead of being used to digest food, a portion of them is absorbed intact into the blood stream and supports the work of the metabolic enzymes. Protease helps the immune system by digesting bacteria, parasites, partially digested protein particles and other toxins. It is also capable of playing a role in neutralizing inflammations. The enzymes amylase and lipase play a part in digesting some viruses as well as healing allergic eruptions of the skin.

Other food enzymes, such as bromelain and papain, although useful in some conditions, work best in a temperature range much higher than that of the human body. This is one reason why concentrated plant enzymes are preferable.

**Pancreatic enzymes:** These enzymes are of animal origin, usually beef or pork. They are the enzymes normally secreted by the pancreas, processed under low heat. They are only active in a very alkaline pH range, such as is found in the normal small intestine. An incompetent digestive tract may not be able to produce this narrow pH range. Nevertheless, these enzymes are extremely helpful in allergic conditions. They play an active role in decreasing inflammation and stopping adverse reactions to food. They are usually given after a meal and sometimes between meals, when inflammation and/or pain is present.

**Antioxidant enzymes:** These enzymes are not used to digest food. Instead, they convert damaging free radicals to oxygen and water, rendering them harmless to the body. They help protect the body from the effects of ionizing radiation and rancid fats. Antioxidant enzymes also appear to participate in breaking apart immune complexes lodged in the body as a result of allergic reactions. Thus, they also help to reduce inflammation in the tissues.

Antioxidant enzymes are produced from plants, mostly sprouts, under a low heat process. The main antioxidant enzymes found in capsules are superoxide dismutase, catalase, glutathione peroxidase and methionine reductase.

The types and amounts of enzymes needed in allergic conditions depend upon the severity of the allergy. An average program would supplement two capsules of plant enzymes before each meal and two capsules of pancreatin after meals. If symptoms develop after the meal, more enzymes may be given. Pancreatic enzyme therapy is effective in controlling pain reactions from kinin-mediated inflammation that sometimes develops in the intestine usually from 15 minutes to two hours after the meal.

Enzymes help in the healing of the intestines and normalization of digestive function in several ways:

1. They ensure proper digestion of food.
2. They take stress off the digestive organs and help "rest" them.
3. They prevent further allergic reactions which can damage the intestinal tissue.

## Step Four:
*Building the immune system.*

Taking a nutrient formula to build the immune system helps speed up healing. A good immune building formula will contain vitamins A, C and E, minerals such as zinc and selenium, glandulars such as thymus and lymph and herbs such as echinacea. Especially with Candida overgrowth the tissue content of vitamin A is often low. (See page 180 for additional nutritional considerations.)

## Step Five:
*Professional care.*

Many forms of chiropractic adjustment techniques not only work to correct structural and neurological dysfunctions, but some types of "non-force" adjusting appear to correct the energetic balance of the body as well. The result is a better-integrated functioning of the body as a whole.

Chiropractors using these techniques are often helpful in recommending appropriate nutritional supplements and enzymes. For severe allergic conditions, professional help is recommended. You may obtain a referral through the directory listed in the appendix.

## Step Six:
### *Healing techniques and dietary follow-up.*

**Homeopathy:** Desensitization and neutralization of allergy is frequently assisted by the use of homeopathic preparations which are minute dilutions of specific substances. These preparations, in liquid or tablet form, are generally taken under the tongue. In the case of allergy, the diluted substance would be an allergen. Because the allergen has been diluted over and over during preparation, the remedy is completely safe and easy to administer. Coffee should not be taken when the allergic individual is under treatment, as it can interfere with the action of the homeopathic preparation.

Homeopathic remedies work well on all types of allergy. They are helpful with food allergens as well as with airborne allergens such as dust, pollen, grass and mold, and with allergies to dogs, cats and horses. They can be added into the program from the start or at any other time. Their action appears to be increased after the allergic individual is detoxified. For this reason, they are useful for allergies which are still active after parasites are under control and the digestive tract has had time to heal. However, particularly for airborne allergies and Candida, they can be very helpful from the start of the program.

**Inhalation Therapy:** It is interesting to note that many "inhalant" allergies are eliminated when proper diet, improvement of digestion and enzyme therapy are employed. On occasions when improvement does not occur as expected, there is special help for stubborn inhalant allergies. When sinus symptoms persist, fungus lodged in the sinuses is often the reason. When fungus is present, tea tree oil (Melaleuca) can be used to speed up healing. Put five to ten drops of tea tree oil in a basin of hot water. Then, breathing through the nose inhale the steam deeply and expel through the mouth. This should be done twice daily for three days. Four to five breaths at a

177

time is sufficient. Tea tree oil comes from Australia, where there are over three hundred known species of tea trees. It has gained popularity recently for its anti-fungal properties.

**Dietary Follow-Up:** Except for the severest cases, the allergic individual should be symptom-free in approximately six weeks when the first six steps have been followed. Damaged tissues may still be healing, however, so precautions should be taken.

If a person returns to his old habits, old problems tend to come back. Once a person is allergy-free, he generally does not want to do things that will cause a return of the condition.

After returning the healthful foods to the diet, the person should continue to take plant enzymes before meals, especially when cooked foods are consumed. This supplies the missing enzymes from those foods and helps to keep digestion competent. The only other supplement that may be needed is a good vitamin and mineral formula, again, because foods tend to be lacking in nutrients. A diet of 70 percent fresh raw fruits, vegetables, seeds and nuts and 30 percent grains, eggs and meat is recommended to prevent the return of allergy.

## Step Seven:
### *Think wellness and wholeness.*

No allergy program would be complete without focusing attention on the importance of the body-mind connection. When allergy arises, it is easy to view the world as a hostile place where hidden dangers lurk. One can become anxious and wary about all sorts of environmental toxins and food ingredients in a supreme effort to protect oneself. While increased awareness of these matters is often necessary to recover from allergy, over-concern is not.

You cannot avoid all environmental poisons and food toxins. Therefore, avoid the "big stuff." Your new knowledge has increased your awareness of major sources of toxicity so that you may now choose to eliminate them from your environment. In doing so, you unburden your healing system. A normal, healthy person is not overly concerned with each chemical he comes in contact with: his body automatically neutralizes and eliminates these chemicals when his tolerance level is not exceeded. Thus, no symptoms occur.

When you have followed the first six steps for six weeks, your body is on a healing course. The minute amount of allergen that once created agonizing symptoms will no longer have that power. Your tolerance will have increased and will continue to increase until your body has normalized and healed.

Once you have put the healing steps in motion and have established the habits necessary to carry them out, it is time to mentally relax. Anxiety itself is known to block healing. If you are experiencing anxiety, depression or any other negative feeling, deliberately think of a happy or positive thought. While you think this positive thought, your brain will begin to produce hormones which will bring forth the feeling. Rest assured that your body now has what it needs to continue healing to the normal state.

Mentally, allergy no longer concerns you. It is time to stop thinking about allergy and to think only wellness and wholeness. Each day becomes a new discovery of your body's increased ability to deal with its environment. Discovery of these new strengths feeds your excitement and adds to your belief that you are whole and well. As you continue your thoughts of wholeness and wellness, your beliefs become *knowing*.

**The Seven Steps** are a basic program for the average person with allergies. In more severe cases, professional care is advised as there are many specialized alternate therapies that may speed the course of healing. Also, if you suspect allergies, or do not know the cause of your symptoms, or do not know to what you are allergic, you should seek professional advice. This is especially true when parasites are present as they can be difficult to detect.

Another reason for seeking outside help is to determine your individual nutrient requirements. In the hundreds of cases of allergy I have treated, no two have been identical, and no two programs have been exactly the same. All, however, have revolved around the basic program of detoxification, checking for pathological organisms, enzyme therapy, nutrients to build the immune system and normalizing the nerve and energetic pathways of the body.

## Additional Nutritional Considerations

**Food Combining:** Most people with allergy have a compromised digestive tract, whether they are aware of it or not. Even when no symptoms in the digestive area are apparent, the ability to digest food is often inadequate, causing allergic symptoms to arise in other areas of the body. Properly combined food takes stress off the digestive tract and allows for more efficient digestion. When food is digested completely, the particles do not become allergens.

Properly combined food requires less enzymes for digestion. In an allergic person, the vital function of enzyme production is compromised. When food is combined properly, less stress is imposed on the digestive tract allowing it time to recover and again function optimally. Enzyme stores then have a chance to build up, and improved digestion prevents allergic reactions from taking place.

There are many food combining charts available on the market today. Many are very complex, explaining the ideal combining methods. In severe allergic cases, this is helpful. However, for the average person with allergies, a modified combining method is sufficient. The most important points of proper food combining, which have worked well in hundreds of clinical cases of allergy, are:

1. Eat all fruit alone, without any other type of food for at least one hour before and one hour after ingestion of the fruit.
2. Meat and other protein can be eaten with any vegetables except the starchy ones such as potato, yam and corn.
3. Whole grains can be eaten with any kind of vegetable including starchy ones.
4. Never follow a protein meal with any kind of sugar dessert, including fruit. When these are eaten together, they cannot be digested thoroughly. This invites not only allergic reactions, but toxins are formed in the intestines which can then be absorbed, stressing the liver and immune system.

**Nutritional Deficiencies:** Nutrition and allergy interact in several ways. Some individuals may have trouble meeting all their nutritional requirements because they have been forced to eliminate many foods (their allergenic foods) from their diet. Also, since people with food allergies have digestive enzyme problems, they have diffi-

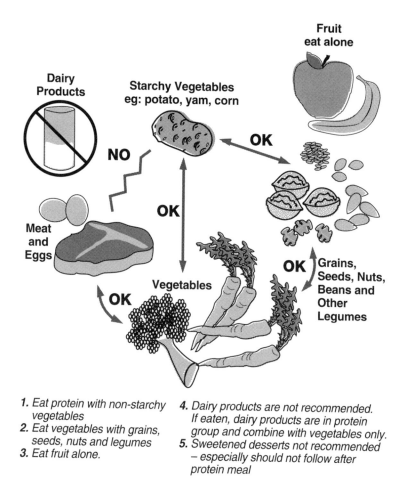

**Fruit**
**eat alone**

**Dairy Products**

**Starchy Vegetables**
**eg: potato, yam, corn**

**NO**

**OK**

**OK**

**Meat and Eggs**

**OK**

**Vegetables**

**OK**

**OK**

**Grains, Seeds, Nuts, Beans and Other Legumes**

1. Eat protein with non-starchy vegetables
2. Eat vegetables with grains, seeds, nuts and legumes
3. Eat fruit alone.

4. Dairy products are not recommended. If eaten, dairy products are in protein group and combine with vegetables only.
5. Sweetened desserts not recommended – especially should not follow after protein meal

*Figure 8.* **Food Combining**

culty breaking down and digesting certain foods. They thereby fail to obtain the nutrients they need.

Some people with allergic problems have special individual biochemical requirements for more of certain vitamins and minerals. Continued allergic stresses on the biochemical system nearly always cause nutritional imbalances or deficiencies. There are many nutrients which benefit allergy. Certainly all of the nutrients known to support the immune system are helpful in allergic conditions. Some of the key nutrients especially helpful are:

**Vitamin C:** Vitamin C appears to act as a natural antihistamine. Large doses of eight grams or more have been known to break an allergic reaction in four to five hours.

Researchers at the Methodist Hospital in Brooklyn studied four hundred people with blood levels low in vitamin C and high in histamine. These people were given 1,000 mg of vitamin C daily. It was found that the histamine levels of the blood dropped, and improvement was seen in the allergic symptoms.

Citrus bioflavonoids, which are actually part of a complete vitamin C, enhance its utilization. Studies done on animals have shown that citrus bioflavonoids may favorably alter the body's metabolism of vitamin C, raising the concentration of the nutrient in certain tissues and enhancing its availability to the body.

The bioflavonoid curcumin appears to have greater anti-inflammatory action than cortisone. Another bioflavonoid, quercitin, prevents the formation of the inflammatory leukotrienes. It also reduces the release of histamine. Even though vitamin C and the bioflavonoids are discussed separately, best results are obtained when they are used together as nature intended.

Vitamin C works more effectively when accompanied by B-complex vitamins, especially pantothenic acid. Without adequate amounts of pantothenic acid, the adrenal hormone cortisone cannot be produced. Natural cortisone relieves and lessens the duration of the allergic reactions.

**$B_6$:** Another vitamin known to have antihistamine effects is vitamin $B_6$, which is extremely important to numerous enzyme systems in the body. As little as 2.5 mg is enough under most circumstances to achieve an anti-histamine effect. Raw liver capsules or tablets also exert an anti-histamine effect on the body.

**Essential Fatty Acids:** The essential fatty acids, LA and LNA, are known powerful inhibitors of inflammation. This is because they are essential for the production of prostaglandins which in turn regulate inflammation. Of these, fresh pressed, unrefined flaxseed oil is probably the best choice. Flaxseed oil contains the highest proportion of Omega 3 and also contains some Omega 6. Fish oil is a good source of Omega 3 in the form of EPA. However, flaxseed oil has the advantages of being better tasting, from a vegetable source and less expensive, and not containing toxins often found in fish.

GLA (gamma-linoleic acid) from evening primrose oil is another nutrient that inhibits the inflammatory response. It has been shown to be effective for people with a history of allergy and eczema.

EPA (eicosapentaenoic acid) from fish oil displaces arachidonic acid in the cell membranes, leaving less arachidonic acid available for inflammatory reactions.

**Minerals:** Minerals are necessary to build enzyme systems. Three minerals especially important to the allergic individual are zinc, selenium and magnesium.

Zinc is perhaps the most vital immune mineral. Without enough zinc, many of the lymph tissues actually shrink, including the thymus and the lymph nodes. The concentration of zinc in the cells affects how energetically the white blood cells attack invaders. Studies show how low zinc levels reduce the number of T-cells. Zinc is important in skin problems and for immune system integrity. When combined with vitamins A, C and E and essential fatty acids, zinc can help speed the healing of eczema.

More recently, research has uncovered the connection of zinc to essential fatty acid metabolism, demonstrating zinc to be crucial to the conversion of some of the nutritionally-derived, essential fatty acids to their active form.

Deficiency of selenium results in diminished resistance to all types of infection, lowered antibody formation and reduced ability of the immune system T-cells to destroy foreign invaders. Supplementation with selenium has been shown to reverse these problems.

Magnesium participates in numerous reactions related to the competence of the immune system, including growth and transformation of B-lymphocytes and the process of protein synthesis whereby immunoglobulins are formed. In clinical studies, magnesium is frequently found to be deficient in allergic individuals.

**Vitamin A:** A lack of vitamin A will cause atrophic changes (wasting away)in the thymus gland and spleen. Vitamin A acts to eliminate free radicals before they can do severe cell damage, thus strengthening the immune system. Researchers have found that children with low vitamin A had abnormally low levels of T-cells in their blood. Vitamin A makes T-cells more active and stronger.

**Vitamin E:** Physicians at Cornell University have demonstrated that vitamin E stimulates antibody production. It helps the T-cells to react faster and more strongly, increasing resistance to disease. As an antioxidant, vitamin E is capable of deactivating free radicals before they can destroy cells.

There are over fifty crucial immune nutrients, and they must be in precise balance for the immune system to work powerfully and efficiently. It is important when considering nutritional needs to recognize each person's inborn biochemical individuality. Every person has a metabolic pattern all his own which increases or decreases the need for specific vitamins and minerals. Typically, nutrients are not like medicines directed at specific diseases. Instead, they work together synergistically to promote a healthy metabolism.

# 19

# Popular Questions

**Q:** *Are you saying that I should never eat any cooked food again?*

**Answer:** I am not recommending that you should never eat any cooked food. I am emphasizing the role of raw food in the natural diet. It is important to realize what the differences are between raw and cooked foods, an important one being enzyme content. Since adequate enzyme levels help protect the body from allergic reactions, enzymes become especially important to allergic individuals. I have never had a patient who converted to a totally raw food diet. However, I have had hundreds of patients who have recovered from allergy. By the same token, a raw food diet is not an extreme diet. The totally cooked food diet is actually the extreme diet, as no other organisms on the face of the earth have ever before existed on it.

If your objective is to eliminate allergy and to stay well, strive for a balanced ratio between cooked and raw foods. Changing the diet to 70 percent raw and 30 percent cooked food is adequate to meet this objective. Whenever you eat cooked food, replace those missing enzymes with plant enzyme supplements. When the enzyme content of the diet remains high, allergies will not return.

# Q: *How much of the essential fatty acids LA (Omega 6) and LNA (Omega 3) is required per day?*

**Answer:** While there are no RDAs for LA and LNA established at this time, the fact that these two fatty acids are indispensable for health and life has been substantiated: based on laboratory studies and other evidence, it is believed that the requirement for LA is two percent of daily calories eaten. This is six grams on a 2,500 calorie diet. The requirement for LNA is considered to be one percent of calories eaten or three grams per day. Approximately one tablespoon of flaxseed oil per day will supply enough LNA.

Although a lack of these nutrients results in disease, only small quantities are required to maintain health.

# Q: *Why do you recommend flaxseed oil?*

**Answer:** Flaxseed oil is the highest source of LNA, containing between 50 and 60 percent. This is the essential fatty acid that is deficient in most western diets. In addition, flaxseed oil contains between 15 and 25 percent LA. This means that you can obtain both essential fatty acids from one oil.

The LNA from flaxseed oil incorporates itself into the membranes of the cells of the body and attracts oxygen to the cells. Besides oxygenating the cells, oxygen acts as a barrier to bacteria and viruses.

The whole seed of flax can be ground up and used to top cereals and salads. Flax seed contains all the essential amino acids making it a complete protein. It supplies many vitamins and trace minerals and is an excellent source of fiber.

Flax seed has historically been used to heal digestive ailments. Inflammation of the stomach, intestines and colon have been helped as well as constipation.

# Q: *How should nuts and seeds be eaten?*

**Answer:** Nuts and seeds should be eaten raw. However, they contain substances called enzyme inhibitors. These inhibitors stop the seed from sprouting until conditions are appropriate. For example, wheat found in ancient Egyptian tombs has been sprouted in this century. Enzyme inhibitors are the source of much indigestion when nuts and seeds are eaten raw. In order to inactivate the enzyme inhibitors, seeds and nuts must either be sprouted or cooked. Cooking, however, destroys LA and LNA as well as many enzymes and nutrients.

Nuts and seeds are best soaked in pure water for 12 to 24 hours depending on the kind of seeds or nuts. After soaking, seeds and nuts will have up to twenty times their original enzyme content and the enzyme inhibitors will be inactivated. Grains and beans are most easily digested when they have been soaked for 24 hours before cooking. Since these foods are usually prepared by cooking, they should be consumed in smaller quantities (part of the 30 percent) than raw foods, and the missing food enzymes should be supplemented.

Q: *If allergy is an inflammatory condition, why not just take anti-inflammatory drugs?*

**Answer:** All drugs have undesirable side effects when taken over weeks, months and years. It is better to normalize the underlying condition producing the inflammation.

The body produces its own inflammation fighters to combat allergic inflammation. These substances are proteases, pancreatin, cortisone and prostaglandins. The key is to stimulate your own body processes to produce these substances while simultaneously discouraging allergen/antibody reactions from occurring. The main tool you have to work with is diet.

Q: *I have too much acid in my stomach because my stomach burns whenever I eat. What can I do besides take antacids?*

**Answer:** Burning pain in the stomach is not necessarily a sign of too much acid in the stomach. Studies show that most people over the age of forty actually have too little stomach acid. Both conditions are known to create burning pain in the stomach.

While antacids do stop pain, they also contribute to other undesirable problems. Frequent taking of antacids alkalinizes the stomach which is the only organ in the body that is supposed to be acid. This has the following effects:

187

1. It upsets normal mineral relationships in the body. For example, phosphorus becomes depleted in the blood when antacids containing magnesium hydroxide or aluminum hydroxide are taken. Decreased phosphorus results in lowered absorption of calcium from the intestines.
2. It hinders absorption of calcium and other minerals which require an acid medium for absorption.
3. It shuts down normal digestion in the stomach so that foods may leave the stomach in a partially digested form. Partially digested particles of food stress the pancreas, are absorbed through the intestine to create allergies, and may ferment or putrefy in the lower bowel to create toxins.
4. It stresses the pH balance of the body.

A better approach to alleviating burning stomach pain is the following:

1. Eliminate food allergens from the diet.
2. Eat whole fresh food in its natural form.
3. Use the rules of correct food combining.
4. Do not overeat.
5. Do not take alcohol with meals.
6. Do not follow meals with sweet desserts.
7. Do not eat when sick or emotionally upset.
8. If burning pain occurs, look for the cause and supplement with plant enzymes. Two capsules of plant enzymes may be taken every fifteen minutes until the pain subsides.

Q. *Is frequent eating of small amounts of food throughout the day the best way to eat?*

**Answer:** Frequent eating of small quantities of food will relieve symptoms in some conditions such as hypoglycemia and digestive problems, but may not be the best way to eat for health. Studies with laboratory animals show that frequent eating uses more enzymes. Eating fewer times per day and less food altogether produces healthier animals with longer life spans.

# 20

# Victory over Allergy

*A*s we have seen, allergy is an inflammatory condition in the body. All inflammation comes from four sources: injury, infection, degeneration and allergy. No matter where inflammation occurs, it is nearly all identical. If the immune system can produce inflammation and allergy, then the immune system can also correct it.

To overcome allergy, increased awareness is the key:

1. Increased awareness that allergy can be involved in your symptoms.
2. Increased awareness that you have the power to take control of your health. No one knows the body better than its owner.
3. Increased awareness that faulty digestion is involved in allergy.
4. Increased awareness of your body's electromagnetic properties.
5. Increased awareness of enzymes and their important role in allergy. Enzymes could be called the "rescue remedy" for allergy.

You do not recover from allergy by treating one part of the body or by simply eliminating histamine. You treat allergy by normalizing body functions. The sequence of healing events is best illustrated by the following formula.

natural food = normal digestion= normal biochemistry
= normal energy = normal health = normal body.

No doctor can give you health. Health is a precious gift you give yourself.

# Epilogue

Are you wondering whatever happened to Pete and Al the Allergy? After reading this book, Pete redoubled his efforts to overcome his health difficulties, bringing himself to a higher state of wellness. Pete's immune system responded and booted out Al the Allergy whose last words were, "I'm homeless. Who's next?"

# Resources

There are many doctors located throughout the United States and Canada who are qualified to help with your allergies and allergy-related health problems. To find one of these doctors, contact one of the groups listed below for a referral. These doctors have all been trained in specific adjustment techniques that help balance body systems. They deal with chronic health problems including allergy, and will counsel you toward a healthier lifestyle.

**Total Body Modification** (A total body technique
  originated by Dr. Victor Frank)
1907 E. Foxmore Circle
Sandy, Utah 84092
1 (801) 243-4TBM
1 (801) 571-2411

**International College of Applied Kinesiology**
  (Founded by Dr. George Goodheart)
114 East 1823 Road
Lawrence, Kansas 66046-9236
(913) 542-1801

**Bio-Energetic Synchronization Technique**
  (Originated by Dr. M.T. Morter Jr.)
1000 West Poplar, Suite "B"
Rogers, Arkansas 72751
1 (800) 874-1478 or (501) 631-2749

**Neuro-Emotional Technique**
   (Originated by Dr. Scott Walker)
500 Second Street
Encinitas, California 92024
(619) 753-1533

**Association of Naturopathic Physicians of British Columbia**
204 - 2786 West 16th Avenue
Vancouver, British Columbia V6K 3C4
(604) 732-7070

**Ontario Naturopathic Medicine Association**
60 Berl Avenue
Toronto, Ontario M8Y 3C7
(416) 503-9554

# Bibliography

Aihara, Herman. *Acid and Alkaline*. Oroville, California: George Oshawa Macrobiotic Foundation, 1986.

Allergy Foundation of America. *Allergy Its Mysterious Causes and Modern Treatment*. New York: Grosset & Dunlap, 1967.

Appleton, Nancy, PhD. *Lick The Sugar Habit*. Garden City Park, New York: Avery Publishing Group Inc., 1988.

Appleton, Nancy, PhD. *Healthy Bones*. Garden City Park, New York: Avery Publishing Group Inc., 1991.

Atkins, Robert C., MD. *Dr. Atkins' Health Revolution*. New York: Bantam Books, 1990.

Balch, James F., MD, and Balch, Phyllis A., CNC. *Prescription for Nutritional Healing*. Garden City Park, New York: Avery Publishing Group Inc., 1990.

Becker, Robert O., MD, and Marino, Andrew A., PhD. *Electromagnetism and Life*. Albany, New York: State University of New York Press, 1982.

Becker, Robert O., MD, and Selden, Gary. *The Body Electric*. New York, NY: William Morrow and Company, Inc., 1985.

Becker, Robert O., MD. *Cross Currents*. Los Angelos, California: Jeremy P. Tarcher, Inc., 1990.

Behrman, Richard E., MD, and Vaughan, Victor C. III, MD. *Nelson Textbook of Pediatrics*. Philadelphia, PA: W.B. Saunders Company, 1987.

Bierman, C. Warren, MD, and Pierson, William E., MD. "Disease of the ear." *Journal of Allergy and Immunology*. 81 (May 1988) 1009-1014.

Bland, Jeffrey, PhD. *Digestive Enzymes*. New Canaan, Connecticut: Keats Publishing, Inc., 1983.

Bluestone, Charles D., MD, and Doyle, William J., PhD. "Anatomy and physiology of Eustachian tube and middle ear related to otitis media." *Journal of Allergy and Clinical Immunology*. 81 (May, 1988) 1004-1009.

Bottomley, H.W., MD, FACP. *Allergy; Its Treatment and Care*. New York: Funk & Wagnalls, 1968.

Breneman, James C., MD. *Basics of Food Allergy*. Second Edition. Springfield, Illinois: Charles C. Thomas, Publisher, 1984.

Brostoff, Jonathan, MA, DM, FRCP, and Chalacombe, Stephen JBDS, MRC.

Path. *Food Allergy and Intolerance.* London, England: Bailliere Tindall, 1987.

Brostoff, Dr. Jonathan and Gamlin, Linda. *The Complete Guide to Food Allergy and Intolerance.* New York: Crown Publishers, Inc., 1989.

Burr, Harold Saxton. *Blueprint for Immortality.* Saffron, Walden: The C.W. Daniel Company Limited, 1988.

Budwig, Dr. Johanna. *Flax Oil as a True Aid Against Arthritis, Heart Infarction, Cancer and Other Diseases.* Vancouver, British Columbia: Apple Publishing Company, 1992.

Burton, Benjamin T., PhD, and Foster, Willis R., MD. *Human Nutrition.* New York: McGraw Hill Book Company, 1988.

Cheraskin, E., MD, DMD, Ringsdorf, W.M., Jr., DMD, and Clark, J.W., DDS. *Diet and Disease.* New Canaan, Connecticut: Keats Publishing, Inc., 1968.

Chiaramonte, Lawrence T., Schneider, Arlene T., and Lifshitz, Iiama (edited by). *Food Allergy.* New York, New York: Marcel Dekker, Inc., 1988.

Cocoa, Arthur F., MD. *Familial Nonreagenic Food Allergy.* Springfield, Illinois: Charles C. Thomas, Publisher, 1953.

Crook, William G., MD. *The Yeast Connection.* Jackson, Tennessee: Professional Books, 1984.

Crook, William G., MD. *Help for the Hyperactive Child.* Jackson, Tennessee: Professional Books, 1991.

Day, Charlene A. *The Immune System Handbook.* North York, Ontario: Potentials Within, 1991.

Dickey, Lawrence D., MD, FACS, edited by. *Clinical Ecology.* Springfield, Illinois: Charles C. Thomas, Publisher, 1976.

Erasmus, Udo. *Fats and Oils.* Vancouver, Canada: Alive Books, 1986.

Erasmus, Udo. *Fats That Heal, Fats That Kill.* Vancouver, Canada: Alive Books, 1993.

Fireman, Phillip, MD, and Slavin, Raymond G., MD. *Atlas of Allergies.* New York, New York: Gower Medical Publishing, 1991.

Gerber, Richard, MD. *Vibrational Medicine.* Santa Fe, New Mexico: Bear & Company, 1988.

Goldberger, Emanual, MD, FACP. *A Primer of Water, Electrolyte, and Acid-Base Syndromes,* 7th Edition. Philadelphia, PA: Lea & Febiger, 1986.

Gottschall, Elaine, BA, MSc. *Food and the Gut Reaction.* Kirkton, Ontario: The Kirkton Press, 1990.

Guyton, Arthur C., MD. *Textbook of Medical Physiology,* 7th Edition. Philadelphia, PA: W.B. Saunders Company, 1986.

Halperin, M.L., MD, and Goldstein, Marc B., MD. *Fluid Electrolyte, and*

*Acid-Base Emergencies.* Philadelphia, PA: W.B. Saunders Company, 1988.

Halpern, Seymour L., MD, FACP, FACN. *Clinical Nutrition.* Philadelphia, PA: J.B. Lippincott Company, 1987.

Harris, M. Coleman, MD. *All About Allergy.* Englewood Cliffs, New Jersey: Prentice-Hall, Inc., 1969.

Howell, Dr. Edward *Enzyme Nutrition.* Wayne, New Jersey: Avery Publishing Group Inc., 1985.

Howell, Dr. Edward. *Food Enzymes for Health and Longevity.* Woodstock Valley, Connecticut: Omangod Press, 1980.

Hunt, Douglas, MD. *No More Cravings.* New York, New York.: Warner Books, Inc., 1987.

Igram, Cass, DO. *Who Needs Headaches?* Cedar Rapids, Iowa: Literary Visions Publishing, Inc.

Kamen, Betty, PhD. *Startling New Facts About Osteoporosis.* Novato, CA: Nutrition Encounter, Inc., 1989.

Lawlor, Glenn J., MD, and Fisher, Thomas J., MD, edited by. *Manual of Allergy and Immunology.* Boston/Toronto: Little, Brown and Company, l988.

Lee, Lita, Ph.D. *Radiation Protection Manual.* Sacramento, CA: Spilman Printing, 1990.

Lehninger, Albert L. *Principles of Biochemistry.* New York, New York: Worth Publishers, Inc., 1982

Linder, Maria C., PhD. *Nutritional Biochemistry and Metabolism.* New York, New York: Elsevier Science Publishing Company, Inc., 1985.

Loomis, Howard F. Jr., DC. *Applied Patho-Physiology and Enzyme Nutrition.* Forsyth, MI: 21st Century Nutrition, Inc., 1990

Mandell, Dr. Marshall, and Scanlon, Lynne Waller. *Dr. Mandells 5-Day Allergy Relief System.* New York: Pocket Books, 1980.

Martens, Richard A., MD, and Martens, Sherlyn, MS, RD. *The Milk Sugar Dilemma: Living with Lactose Intolerance.* East Lansing, MI: Medi-Ed Press, 1967.

McDougall, John A., MD, and McDougall, Mary A. *The McDougall Plan.* Piscataway, NJ: New Century Publishers, 1983.

Miller, Martha J., MAT. *Pathophysiology Principles of Disease.* Philadelphia, PA: W.B. Saunders Co., 1983.

Moore, Richard, MD, PhD, and Webb, George D., PhD. *The K Factor.* New York, New York: Pocket Books, 1987.

Morell, Franz, MD. *The Mora Concept.* Heidelberg, Germany: Karl F. Haug Publishers, 1990.

Morter, M.T. Jr., BS, MA, DC. *Correlative Urinalysis*. Rogers, Arkansas: B.E.S.T. Research Inc., 1987.

Morter, Dr. M. Ted Jr. *Your Health Your Choice*. Hollywood, Florida: Fell Publishers, Inc., 1990.

Morter, M.T. Jr., BS, MA, DC. *The Healing Field*. Rogers, Arkansas: B.E.S.T. Research, Inc., 1991.

National Research Council. *Recommended Dietary Allowances, 10th edition*. Washington, DC: National Academy Press, 1989.

Paterson, Barbara. *The Allergy Connection*. Wellingborough, New York: Thorsons Publishers, Ltd., 1985

Patterson, Ray, MD. *Allergic Diseases*. Philadelphia, PA: J.B. Lippincott Company, 1972.

Pennington, Jean A.T., PhD, RD. *Food Values of Portions Commonly Used*. New York, New York: Harper & Row Publishers, Inc. 1989.

Philpott, William H., MD, and Kalita, Dwight K., PhD. *Brain Allergies*. New Canaan, Connecticut: Keats Publishing, Inc., 1980.

Philpott, William H., MD, and Kalita, Dwight K., PhD. *Victory Over Diabetes*. New Canaan, Connecticut: Keats Publishing, Inc., 1983.

Pottenger, Francis M. Jr., MD. *Pottenger's Cats*. La Mesa, California: Price-Pottenger Nutrition Foundation, 1989.

Randolph, Theron G., MD, and Moss, Ralph W., PhD. *An Alternate Approach to Allergies*. New York: Harper & Row, Publishers, 1990.

Rapp, Doris J., MD. *Allergies and Your Family*. New York: Sterling Publishing Co., Inc., 1985.

Roberts, H. J., MD. *Aspartame (NutraSweet*) Is It Safe?* Philadelphia, Pennsylvania: The Charles Press, Publishers, 1990.

Rochlitz, Steven. *Allergies and Candida*. Mahopac, New York: Human Ecology Balancing Sciences, Inc., 1991.

Rowe, Albert H., MD. *Food Allergy*. Springfield, Illinois: Charles C. Thomas, Publisher, 1972.

Rubin, Emanuel, MD, and Farber, John L. MD. *Pathology*. Philadelphia, PA: J.B. Lippincott Company, 1988.

Sampson, Hugh A., MD, and Cooke, Sarak., S.B. "Food allergy and the potential allergenicity-antigenicity of microparticulated egg and cow's milk proteins." *Journal of the American College of Nutrition*. Vol. 9, No. 4, 410-417 (1990).

Santillo, Humbart, BS, MH. *Food Enzymes*. Prescott Valley, Arizona: Hohm Press, 1987.

Schechter, Steven R., ND. *Fighting Radiation and Chemical Pollutants with*

*Foods, Herbs, and Vitamins.* Encinitas, California: Vitality Link, 1990.

Schmidt, Michael A. *Childhood Ear Infections.* Berkeley, California: North Atlantic Books, 1990.

Schwarz, Edward F., PhD. *Endocrines, Organs, and their Impact.* Hales Corners, WI: Cornerstone Press, 1985.

Seldin & Giebish. *The Regulation of Acid-Base Balance.* New York: Raven Press, Ltd., 1989.

Sheinkin, David, MD, Schachter, Michael, MD, and Hutton, Richard. *The Food Connection.* Indianapolis/New York: The Bobbs-Merrill Company, Inc., 1979.

Speer, Frederic, MD. *Food Allergy.* New York: John Wright PSE. Inc., 1983.

Stone, Robert B., PhD. *The Secret Life of Your Cells.* Westchester, PA.: Whitford Press, 1989.

Szekely, Edmond Bordeaux *The Essene Gospel of Peace.* United States: International Biogenic Society, 1981.

Taube, E. Louis, MD. *Food Allergy and the Allergic Patient.* Springfield, Illinois: Charles C. Thomas, Publisher, 1978.

Thompson, W. Grant, MD. *Gut Reactions.* New York/London: Plenum Press, 1989.

Trowbridge, John Parkes, MD, and Walker, Morton, DPM. *The Yeast Syndrome.* Toronto/New York: Bantam books, 1986.

Washton, Arnold, PhD, and Boundy, Donna, MSW. *Willpower's Not Enough.* New York: Harper Collins, Publishers, 1990.

Werbach, Melvyn, R., MD. *Nutritional Influences on Illness.* Tarzana, California: Third Line Press, Inc., 1988.

Werbach, Melvyn, R., MD. *Third Line Medicine.* Guernsey, Channel Islands: The Guernsey Press Co. Ltd., 1986.

Williams, Warwick, Dyson, Bannister. *Gray's Anatomy.* Thirty-Seventh Edition. Edinburgh, London: Churchill Livingstone, 1989.

Wolf, Max, MD, and Ransberger, Karl, PhD. *Enzyme Therapy.* Los Angeles, California: Regent House, 1977.

# Index

## A

acid-base, 65-79, 98, 194-195, 197
acid-base balance, 65-79, 98, 197
acne, 40, 58, 88
addiction, 45, 53-56, 81, 95, 151
Adey, Ross,167
adrenal glands, 48-49
alcohol, 12, 22, 53-55, 59, 87-88,
    95-96, 113-114, 123, 126, 149-
    151, 155, 188
alginates, 149
allergens, 7, 9, 11-12, 15-18, 23, 25-
    26, 31-37, 43, 45-51, 55, 61-62,
    82-83, 89, 111, 115-116, 119,
    135-137, 144, 146, 150, 164,
    170, 174, 177, 179-180, 187-
    188, 197
allergic-like, 16-17, 56, 108
allergic load, 24-25
almonds, 70, 73, 116, 129-130
amnesia, 39
amylase, 92-93, 96-98, 140, 175
anaphylaxis, 7, 36-37
anemia, 40, 136
angina pectoris, 40
antacids, 28, 35, 72, 86, 98, 111,
    115, 187-188
antibiotics, 35, 44, 58, 61-63, 127,
    137-138, 140, 143-144, 146
antibodies,9, 13, 16-17, 31-34, 36,
    42, 44, 50, 59, 63, 89, 108, 138-
    139, 183-184, 187
antihistamines, 5, 18, 182
antioxidant enzymes, 175-176
apathy, 39
aphasia, 39
apples, 47, 73, 130, 133, 193-194
apricots, 73
arachidonic acid, 121, 124-125, 183

arthralgia, 40
arthritis, 7-8, 13, 23-24, 27, 40, 46-
    48, 72, 81, 88, 101-102, 194
artichokes, 73, 117, 173
artificial flavors, 149
Aspartame, 149, 196
Aspirin, 10, 28, 35, 37, 48, 147, 151
asthma, 4-5, 7, 10, 22, 40, 48, 63,
    72, 88, 100, 126, 135, 138, 147-
    149
Atkins, Robert C., MD, 27, 193
atopic, 17, 138
avocados, 73, 117, 127, 132-133

## B

backaches, 23, 41
Backster, Cleve, 154-155
Baker, Dr. Robin, 161
bananas, 23, 73, 93-94, 130, 147
barley, 74, 130, 150
beans, 70, 73, 106, 117, 127, 187
Beasley, Joseph D. MD, 81
Becker, Robert O., MD, 159-161,
    164-166, 193
bed-wetting, 13, 24, 41, 61, 135,
    141-144
beef, 11, 67, 70, 74, 82, 142, 175
belching, 40, 64, 82
benzoic acid, 149
berries, 73, 130-131
BHA, 147
BHT, 147
biochemical individuality, 9, 184
birth control pills, 35, 58-60
blackouts, 39
bleeding, 40, 126, 136
bloating, 40, 60, 64, 98-99, 114
bread, 55, 73, 98, 125, 143, 150
breast feeding, 137-139, 149

# About the Author

D r. Carolee Bateson-Koch completed her basic science requirements at Fresno State College in California before entering the
Los Angeles College of Chiropractic. She received her Doctor of Chiropractic degree in 1968, graduating as valedictorian of her class. Dr.
Bateson-Koch has continued postgraduate studies, earning a PhD in
nutrition. In 1988, she received her Doctor of Naturopathy degree
from the Ontario College of Naturopathy in Canada and was hon-
ored with the nutrition award for her graduating class.

Dr. Bateson-Koch's special interest in the treatment of allergy
with use of nutrition and natural therapies developed as she realized
that allergic reactions were underlying many common conditions
seen in her office. Through writing and lecturing, she is committed
to elevating both community and professional awareness of the scope
of allergic conditions and their effective treatment.

Dr. Bateson-Koch has traveled throughout the United States,
Canada, China, Germany and Australia gathering information on
safe and useful therapies for allergy. She currently resides and practices chiropractic in Alberta, Canada. Dr. Bateson-Koch is an active
member of the Alberta College of Chiropractors, and the Canadian
Chiropractic Association. She is a member of the Governor's Club of
the Canadian Memorial Chiropractic College.

# Other titles by Alive Books

**Fats That Heal Fats That Kill**
*The complete guide to fats, oils, cholesterol and human health.*
Udo Erasmus, 480 pp softcover

**Healing with Herbal Juices**
*A practical guide to herbal juice therapy: nature's preventative medicine.*
Siegfried Gursche, 240 pp softcover

**Silica – The Forgotten Nutrient**
*Healthy skin, shiny hair, strong bones, beautiful nails. A guide to the vital role of organic vegetal silica in nutrition, health, longevity and medicine.*
Klaus Kaufmann, 128 pp softcover

**Silica – The Amazing Gel**
*An essential mineral for radiant health, recovery and rejuvenation.*
Klaus Kaufmann, 176 pp softcover

**The Joy of Juice Fasting**
*For health, cleansing and weight loss.*
Klaus Kaufmann, 114 pp softcover

**Making Sauerkraut and Pickled Vegetables at Home**
*The original lactic acid fermentation method.*
Annelies Schoeneck, 80 pp softcover

**Cancer – There is Hope**
*Alternative treatments, testimonials of cures, the Essiac story and more.*
Byrun F. Tylor, 128 pp softcover

**Devil's Claw Root and Other Natural Remedies for Arthritis**
Rachel Carston, 128 pp softcover

**International Health News Yearbook (Annual)**
*The latest, most important discoveries in nutrition, health and medicine.*
Hans Larsen, 96 pp softcover

All books are available at your local health food store or from
Alive Books, PO Box 80055 Burnaby BC V5H 3X1